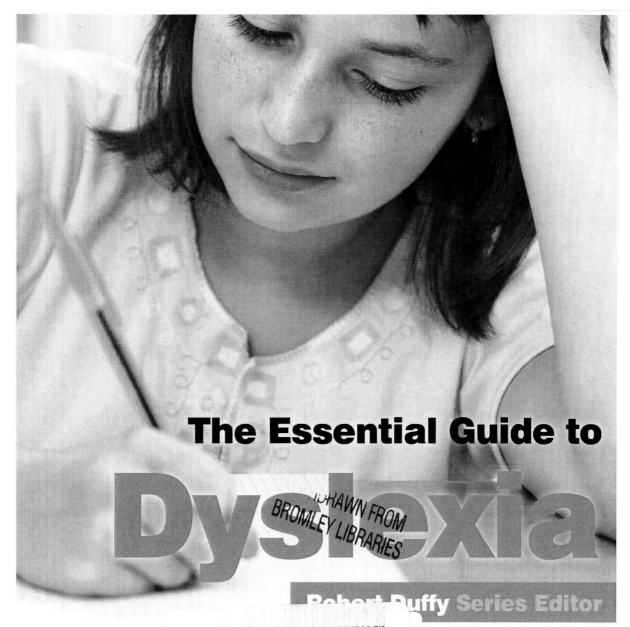

The Essential Guide to

Dyslexia

Robert Duffy Series Editor

Published in Great Britain in 2018 by
need2know
Remus House
Coltsfoot Drive
Peterborough
PE2 9BF
Telephone 01733 898103
www.need2knowbooks.co.uk
All Rights Reserved
© Need2Know
SB ISBN 978-1-91084-374-1
Cover photograph: Dreamstime

Contents

Introduction

Every weekday, millions of kids get up and go to school. It's highly common for parents to feel some sort of loss when their kids start school, but the vast majority of those kids will work their way through the mainstream educational system with very few issues from start to finish. These are the children whose anxiety is outweighed by their eagerness to absorb all of the information and experiences available, and whose personalities and mental skills properly suit them to conventional schooling.

One child might take years to master an educational skill like reading or writing while others may appear to get it down in a few weeks. Some kids can already read before they even start school. However, for some kids education can be a real uphill battle, and in some of these cases that can be due at least in part to learning difficulties. These difficulties can sometimes become apparent just a few months after starting school: they are struggling to fit in, to keep up with their classmates, to pick up the information each lesson is meant to impart.

For these children, the best way is often to go down the route of special education, but that can take a whole lot of time, money and bureaucracy. It can take several years to get your child the support they need. In the meantime, everyday another comparison is waiting to be drawn between your child and their peers. Maybe the other kids run out of school covered in "Well Done!" stickers while your child remains undecorated.

If the teacher doesn't know what's holding your child back, it's easy for them to assume it's down to a lack of effort. Maybe your child has been on the same reading book for a month, while the others have moved on. It can be difficult to make these observations without feeling bad for "judging" your child. It can be difficult not to wonder if this is because of something you've done wrong. But your child's difficulty can be as a result of a number of different factors, including…

- Writing, arithmetic and reading;
- Mental or physical disabilities;
- Health and medical issues;
- Behavioural or emotional issues;
- Hearing, vision or speaking.

In many cases, the differences between your child and their peers will be fairly obvious after just a short period of schooling. These difficulties can be a major source of stress not only for the parent, but for the child who is constantly falling behind their peers, losing self esteem and maybe even getting bullied. Sometimes talking to a teacher can be helpful, while other times you can get a weak response of "They'll catch up."

A parent can often already be at breaking point by the time they've asked for help, so this won't be what they're looking for. The longer it takes to figure things out, the worse things might seem. The relationships between you, your child and their teacher can become strained. Rather than properly addressing your concern, a teacher might simply label you a helicopter parent and feel that you simply aren't taking responsibility for your child's lack of motivation (which, in fairness to teachers, is not unheard of).

The school can become a stressful battleground. At this stage, you may begin to wonder what your legal rights are, and where you should be going for help. It can become clear that if you'd known what to do sooner, things could have been sorted out much more easily. Do you know how to access the various publications and associations that exist to help parents like you?

The aim of this book is to provide all of this information in a clear and easy way.

Note to the Reader

This book provides general information on dyslexia and other learning difficulties, but should not be used in the place of professional advice. It can be a very helpful guide to use alongside your doctor's advice. If you have any concerns about yourself or your child or whether or not either of you have dyslexia, please talk to your GP.

While every care has been taken to ensure that the information in this text is accurate, the author does not claim to have the proper qualifications to diagnose this condition. Please talk to your doctor before undertaking any form of treatment.

Knowing There's an Issue

Lots of parents will notice pretty quickly if their child has a problem. Always being at the bottom of the class, not understanding what's happening or knowing the answer and not being able to share the information can be very upsetting for a child. This can make it all the more upsetting when the people you go to refuse to acknowledge that there's an actual problem, instead insisting that your kid is simply unmotivated, won't listen, is slow or naughty.

Eventually, you might even end up believing them. It's difficult to know what to do in these situations. Surely, if you really love your child, you can just accept they won't do well and leave everyone alone? Surely degrees and awards aren't the most important things in life?

And you're right: education isn't the most important thing. But getting your child the same opportunities that everyone else has is still very important.

One common concern is that if you keep "nagging" the teachers, the resulting resentment could negatively alter the way they treat your child. Approaching the headteacher of the school can eventually lead to the same concerns. Nobody wants their kid to get unfair treatment as a result of their own actions. So who should you be talking to?

Struggling with the Smallest Challenges

If your child can't read, it's likely they won't be able to recognise their own name on labels and badges. This can make things really difficult in primary school, where many items are labelled to make sure they aren't lost or stolen.

Your child's difficulties will create unexpected challenges even when they aren't trying to do classwork or homework.

What is a "Statement"?

In more proactive schools, teachers may spot your child's struggles before you do and will contact you about it. They may suggest putting a statement on your child. While this may sound alarming, it simply means placing a Statement of Educational Needs on your child. This is where a problem is formally identified so that the school and other professionals can be alerted to arrangements that need made. We'll talk about this in greater detail in Chapter Twelve: Help is at Hand!. This is especially common if the school are aware that your child has another sibling or siblings with learning difficulties.

If you work closely with the school, this Statement of Educational Needs should come through fairly quickly, but it is possible for it to take a number of years.

Dyslexia, Dyspraxia and Dyscalculia in Children

Early Identification Checklist

If your pre-school child has dyslexia, they may have some or all of these difficulties. While many are common in children for a time, if your child hasn't grown out of them by the time most of their peers have, it may be an indication that support is needed.

Weaknesses

☐ Does your family have a history of learning difficulties?

☐ Does your child have difficulties putting shoes on the right feet, tying laces, buttons or getting dressed?

☐ Are you often told your child is not paying attention or making an effort?

☐ Does your child trip over and knock things down a lot?

☐ Does your child tend to confuse colour names (e.g. calling red yellow)?

☐ Does your child tend to confuse directions (e.g. up/down and left/right)?

☐ Can your child put things in order (e.g. days of the week, the alphabet, months of the year)?

☐ Does your child tend to hold pens and pencils too tightly?

☐ Can they follow instructions, such as putting four beads in order by colour?

☐ Are they able to pick the odd word out from lists (e.g. dog, fog, cat, bog)?

☐ Do they struggle with labels and thinking of words?

☐ Can they clap a rhythm back to you?

☐ Do they struggle with games like hopping, catching and skipping?

☐ Does your child show no interest in books, but still enjoy listening to stories?

☐ Is your child lisping, struggling to speak clearly or not speaking at all?

Strengths

☐ Does your child have a lot of original, quick thoughts?

☐ Is your child particularly good at construction games such as building, keyboards, remote controls and LEGO?

☐ Do they seem intelligent but still struggle with minor tasks?

☐ Are they good at arts and crafts?

Children's Checklist

Once your child reaches school age, dyslexia may become apparent in different ways. If you believe there is cause for concern and your child is exhibiting some of the following issues, you may wish to get support.

Reading and Spelling

When your child is reading and writing, do they…

☐ Get confused between letters that look similar (u and n, m and n, etc)?

☐ Read words backwards (now becomes won, dab becomes bad)?

☐ Read the same word right sometimes but wrong other times?

☐ Get confused between short words like for, from and of?

☐ Read well, but without understanding what they're reading?

☐ Frequently lose their place and struggle to re-find it?

☐ Rearrange sentences ("the cat sat on the mat" becomes "the mat sat on the cat")?

☐ Rearrange letters (felt becomes left)?

☐ Get confused between letters that sound similar, like f, th and v?

Writing

Despite being told several times, does your child still…

☐ Not know if they write with their left or right hand?

☐ Forget to cross 't's and dot 'i's?

☐ Write in a slope, even with guide lines and margins?

☐ Leave out paragraphs and punctuation, or use them in the wrong places?

☐ Struggle to draw numbers and letters?

☐ Put capital letters in the wrong places or leave them out entirely?

Other Indications

☐ Does your family have a history of dyslexia or similar issues?

☐ Does your child have difficulty concentrating or resisting distractions?

☐ Does your child struggle with sequences such as nursery rhymes, numbers in tables, months of the year, days of the week?

☐ Does your child have difficulties telling the time?

☐ Does your child have problems with their short term memory when it comes to instructions and written phrases?

☐ Does your child have problems copying things from the blackboard?

☐ Is your child unable to follow multiple instructions at once?

☐ Do they have an inability to use telephone directories and thesauruses?

☐ Do they tend to confuse maths symbols like divide and multiply?

☐ Do they tend to use either their right or left eyes/hands in certain tasks (this is called mixed laterality)?

☐ Do they have problems with tasks like tying shoelaces?

☐ Do they hold their pen awkwardly/too tightly?

☐ Do they confuse directions, such as east/west, over/under, up/down, in/out?

☐ Were they a "late bloomer"?

Dyscalculia Checklist

Does your child have issues with…

☐ memorising multiplication tables?

☐ estimating numbers: tens, hundreds, thousands?

☐ working out averages?

☐ understanding things like carrying, borrowing and place value?

☐ working out the speed in miles per hour?

☐ learning the date?

☐ describing how they got the answer to a mathematical problem?

☐ limited strategic planning such as games like chess?

☐ telling the time and related concepts like days, weeks and seasons?

☐ understanding $2+5=7$ and $5+2=7$?

☐ understanding fractions?

☐ working out percentages?

☐ working out simple money and change?

Does your child…

- ☐ get confused between numbers, e.g. 42 and 24?
- ☐ confuse minus, subtract and take away?
- ☐ confuse add, plus and add on?
- ☐ reverse or transpose numbers when writing and reading?

Dyspraxia Checklist

The following issues are common indicators that your child might have dyspraxia. Please remember that when a child is only starting school, it's common to make any number of these mistakes. Advice only needs to be sought if your child continues to exhibit these symptoms after all of their peers have grown out of them. Not every child who's a little clumsy or takes their time with things should automatically be labelled as dyspraxic.

Infants

Delayed milestones that might be exhibited by very young children include issues with…

- ☐ Sleeping;
- ☐ Falling over when trying to sit up;
- ☐ Delayed start to walking;
- ☐ Eating messily;
- ☐ Lifting small objects;
- ☐ Baby puzzles or building blocks;
- ☐ Talking late and having speech problems;
- ☐ "Bum shuffling" rather than crawling;
- ☐ Fidgeting and worrying.

Children

Later issues might include…

☐ Constant fidgeting;

☐ Fiddling with hands and other items, swinging legs;

☐ Spilling drinks;

☐ Frequently bumping into things;

☐ Falling over for no obvious reason;

☐ Struggling to balance on one leg or on tiptoe;

☐ Struggling to tie shoelaces;

☐ Have problems telling the time;

☐ Have problems dressing and doing up buttons;

☐ Have problems using stairs and steps;

☐ Stumbles into doors;

☐ Have problems using knives and forks;

☐ Knocks things over;

☐ Never sits still.

Difficulties during play can include…

☐ Issues with fine motor skills;

☐ Using craft tools, e.g. scissors;

☐ Struggling to thread needles;

☐ Hitting moving balls, as in rounders or tennis;

☐ Roller skating;

☐ Difficulties with coordination when swimming;

☐ Riding a bike;

☐ Catching or kicking a ball;

☐ Painting and colouring small areas;

☐ Puzzles, construction games, LEGO, etc.

Difficulties during class and in other formal settings might include…

☐ Frequently losing their place while reading;

☐ Changing writing hand regularly, not knowing which hand to write with;

☐ Inability or refusal to use margins;

☐ Struggling to copy symbols such as squares, triangles and rectangles;

☐ Inability to follow instructions;

☐ They have difficulty reading maps;

☐ They have difficulty copying work from whiteboards, etc.;

☐ Their writing slopes on the page;

☐ Writes in different directions on the same paper;

☐ When writing, grips the pencil very tightly and awkwardly.

Contacting an Educational Psychologist

One step you might consider taking at this stage is to find out who the educational psychologist is for your area and get in touch. It's probably best if you at least let your child's school know this is happening, as unexpected classroom visits can be pretty disruptive! After talking to you, it's likely they will go to your child's school in order to carry out the necessary tests.

This can seem a little daunting, but don't worry! The tests aren't scary, and will allow the psychologist either to confirm your suspicious or put them to bed, and either of these options is better than being left in the dark. If it turns out that your child has dyslexia, a plan of action will be needed as soon as possible to stop them from falling any further behind their classmates.

While it may sometimes seem a little extreme to contact a psychologist without going through your child's school, this can often be the best plan of action. Many schools are reluctant to call in professionals unless it's completely unavoidable, and learning difficulties are best worked with if they're identified early on. It's also an important move for your child's self confidence, as it can be easy for undiagnosed learning difficulties to make a child believe they are simply a bit thick.

Once the written report from your educational psychologist arrives, there can be a whole new hurdle to deal with: figuring out what it actually means and what you can do to help. For example, some reports might conclude that a child has SpLDs ("specific learning difficulties") – these fall under the heading of "dyslexia". Not everyone will automatically know what that means! You'll need to get an understanding of what your child's school is obligated to help with. You'll also need to find out what sort of support is available and how you can access it.

Another option for having your child assessed is to have it carried out by specialist teachers with the goal of identifying the child's specific areas of strength and weakness. In either case, once the report is completed, an IED (Individual Education Plan) can be created and put in place for your child.

There's also the issue of whether or not you live in a county where the psychologist service will put dyslexia on reports. While many include it by now, there are still a handful of counties that haven't got there yet.

When it comes to finding out this type of information, your local library may well be the best place to check. The things and people you find there can be invaluable. The staff there will be well versed in helping people find the resources they need, especially if they've worked there for a number of years.

Another group you may consider contacting is the British Dyslexia Association. Often local branches of the Association will be able to offer your child a place which will allow them to attend weekly classes to support their learning. The people who run these groups are all dedicated to helping children like yours, and have a great amount of experience in this field. Giving your child the opportunity to learn surrounded by other children with the same learning difficulties can not only boost their learning skills but also their confidence as they will see that they are not alone.

One thing you need to know is that while some schools may claim a child must be moved to a "special school" if they receive a Statement for Education, this isn't correct and goes against what the Department of Education says. While you and your child may decide that changing schools is the best option for your situation, most children actually stay in their original school.

At the end of the day, there really is a light at the end of the tunnel. It's more than possible for your child with dyslexia to excel and reach an average or above-average level in many areas of education. They'll get there, just don't give up! It's very common for parents of children with learning difficulties to feel isolated, but there are so many resources available if you know where to look.

Screening

Some of the tests that might be worth considering for your child include…

Age	Name of Test/Screening
Children	Lucid – Memory Booster – Memory Training for Children
3-6:11 years	Phonological Pipa
4:6-6:5 years	Dyslexia Early Screening Test (DEST-2)
4-8 years	Lucid CoPS – Cognitive Profiling System
4-15 years	Lucid Rapid Dyslexia Screening
4-16 years	Lucid Ability – Verbal and Non-Verbal Reasoning
6-14:11 years	Phonological Assessment Battery (PhAB)
6-14+ years	Dyscalculia Screener
6:6-16:5 years	Dyslexia Screening Test Junior (DST-J)
5-7 years	Phonological PAT
5-14 years	Aston Index Assessment
7-14 years	Comprehension Booster – Improve reading and listening comprehension
7-adult	Lucid – ViSS – Visual Stress Screener
8-11 years	LASS – Lucid Assessment System for Schools
11-15 years	LASS – Lucid Assessment System for Schools
11-24 years	Lucid Exact – Computerised Assessment of Literacy
15+ years	LADS Plus – Lucid Adult Dyslexia Screening (Plus Version)
16:5 years+	Dyslexia Adult Screening Test (DAST)
Adult	LADS – Lucid Adult Dyslexia Screening
Any Age	Educational Psychologist Report

These tests are available from a variety of different sources. For example, the 'Dyscalculia' Screener can be accessed through GL-Assessment, while the fully computerised 'Lucid' Screening Systems are accessed through Lucid.

The most detailed test available is the educational psychologist's assessment, which can also check your child's IQ (intelligence quotient). Many universities, colleges and schools allow their pupils to access an educational psychologist for free. However, this can take some time as the psychologist will only be contacted if the school believes your child has a severe, long-term issue.

If you can afford it, it's often a better choice to consult an educational psychologist privately.

The system used to require that in order to access grants, students would have to have an educational psychologist's report carried out every year. However, the rules have since changed and if you've had one after the age of 16 you may never need another one. You can find more information on these rules through the DFE (Department for Education) website.

Importantly, while the system may not insist on your child having additional reports, they may still be beneficial. Assessments can be vital in finding out how much progress has been made and, more importantly, finding out your child's specific needs at the time of testing.

Will the Schools Identify a Problem?

One issue is identifying exactly what qualifies as an SEN (special educational need). This book hopes to discuss some of the invisible conditions that are hard to spot and therefore tricky to assess. Among the most notable is ADHD (attention deficit hyperactivity disorder), which is often misidentified as simple spoiltness or naughtiness.

While one school will be ready to spot an issue early and start to help it as quickly as possibles, others won't have the necessary resources and will instead delay the subject for years in the hopes that the problem will be dealt with by another school when the child eventually moves on. Similarly, there are some LEAs (Local Education Authorities) that are very good at identifying children who are struggling in the first few years of schooling, while others aren't so consistent.

Any Questions?

There may be any number of questions flying through your head right now, such as…

- Where can I find help?
- How should I start searching for information?
- What is dyspraxia?
- What is a Statement of Educational Needs?
- Should a statement be placed on my child?
- What is the Local Education Authority (LEA)?
- What is the Department for Education (DFE)?
- What legal entitlements does my child have?

- Will my child need to change schools?
- What is ADHD (attention deficit hyperactivity disorder)?
- What are dyscalculia, dysgraphia and dyslexia?
- What support is available?

These are the FAQs of parents in your position. While there is an Education Advisory Service run by the government, most parents don't really know about it or where to access it. This service produces a vast amount of booklets on the subject, but the great stack of literature is often more daunting than it is helpful. In fact, in many cases you'd need a pretty high degree of education to be able to make head or tail of the contents of these booklets – and that's if you even manage to find them in the first place.

The aim of this book is to make all of this information available and easy to understand. We hope to explain what support is available to you, and where you can look for the guidance you need. This is not a scientific text on every disorder known to man, but a simple guide to just a few of the more common difficulties we may face.

Famous People with the Gift of Dyslexia

There are loads of accomplished, talented people out there who have dyslexia or related learning difficulties. How many of these lawmakers did you know?

Law & Justice

- David Boies (Attorney)
- Jeffrey H. Gallet (Judge)
- Erin Brockovich (Investigator)

How Many Types of Dyslexia Are There?

We are currently aware of three main types of dyslexia. These are…

Acquired Dyslexia

- Brain damage, trauma, etc (generally permanent);
- Glue ear (temporary);
- Strokes, etc (can be permanent or temporary).

Developmental Dyslexia

- Premature birth;
- Malnutrition in the womb;
- Neglect or abuse;
- Poor nutrition;
- Issues with foetus.

Primary Dyslexia (Deep Dyslexia)

- Family history;
- Damage to cerebral cortex (left-hand side of brain);
- High percentage of left-handedness;
- 75-80% male;
- Linked to chromosomes 6 and 15.

Many children with dyslexia are very clever in many ways but don't seem to reach their full academic potential, despite always asking questions and taking part. A nice quote comes from Princess Beatrice:

Dyslexia is not a pigeonhole to say you can't do anything. It is an opportunity and a possibility to learn differently. You have magical brains, they just process differently. Don't feel like you should be held back by it.

Famous People with the Gift of Dyslexia

There are loads of accomplished, talented people out there who have dyslexia or related learning difficulties. How many of these entertainers did you know?

Actors & Entertainers

- Harry Anderson
- Cher
- Whoopi Goldberg
- Keanu Reeves
- Anthony Hopkins

- Charley Boorman
- Susan Hampshire
- Steven Spielberg
- Loretta Young
- Vince Vaughn
- Christopher Lowell
- Anderson Cooper
- Orlando Bloom
- Jay Leno
- Caitlyn Jenner
- Tom Cruise
- Harry Belafonte

What Have We Learned?

- If you think something needs done to help your child, you're probably right. If you're really concerned, don't allow people to fob you off with lame excuses. Don't be aggressive, but be firm and ask to have the appropriate tests carried out. A full assessment or educational psychologist's report may be necessary.

- Make sure you understand the information you're being given. For example, if you're told your child's "reading level" is 3, ask what that means in terms of reading age so you know where you stand.

2

What Are Special Educational Needs?

Many teachers still function under the understanding that children born into homes where education and reading are valued will automatically perform well in school, and that those who don't do so well have been failed somehow. But as tempting as this theory may be because of its simplistic nature, there simply are some children who don't pick things up as automatically as other kids, and who will need some extra support.

The term "Special Educational Needs" is pretty broad and covers anything from difficulties with sight and hearing to physical and mental handicaps. There are hundreds of thousands of schoolchildren who fit into this category. Interestingly, children who are highly gifted also fall under this category and are similarly often denied the education they deserve for financial reasons.

Essentially, this is a grouping used to describe anyone who doesn't slot perfectly into mainstream education. There are many people out there with learning difficulties that have never been properly recognised. In fact, a great number of children who are simply labelled as "naughty" in school behave this way because they struggle to fit into a system that emphasises actions like watching, listening and sitting quietly.

The fact that these children need more help than is typically provided to the average student creates extra expenses. As a general rule, the government allows for a specific amount of money per child for education, so anyone who falls outside of the norm can be left behind.

Famous People with the Gift of Dyslexia

There are loads of accomplished, talented people out there who have dyslexia or related learning difficulties. How many of these entrepreneurs and business leaders did you know?

Business Heavy Hitters

- Richard Branson (Founder, Virgin Enterprises)
- Lord Sugar (Founder, Amstrad)
- Sir Peter Leitch (New Zealand businessman)
- O.D. McKee (Founder, McKee Foods)
- Dame Anita Roddick (philanthropist, human rights campaigner and entrepreneur, Body Shop)
- Ted Turner (President, Turner Broadcasting Systems)
- Frank W. Woolworth
- Henry Ford
- Robert Woodruff (President, Coca-Cola)
- Charles Schwab (Investor)
- David Neeleman (CEO, jetBlue Airways)
- Sir Norman Foster (Founder, Foster & Partners)
- Ingvar Kamprad (Founder, IKEA)
- John T Chambers (CEO, Cisco Systems)

What Have We Learned?

- A wide range of difficulties can fall under the heading of Special Educational Needs.

- One of the main challenges is identifying the exact cause of the difficulty. Until the problem has been identified, it can be difficult to come up with the best education plan for the child.

- It's very rare for a child with SENs to need to go to a special school. The vast majority of these children will stay in mainstream education with a little extra help.

3

Specific Learning Difficulties – Dyslexia

Confusion is often caused by the fact that SpLDs (Specific Learning Difficulties) and Dyslexia tend to be lumped in under the same umbrella. At this stage, it's widely accepted that dyslexia is just one member of a whole set of difficulties including…

- Dyscalculia;
- Dyspraxia;
- ADHD (Attention Deficit Hyperactivity Disorder);

- ADD (Attention Deficit Disorder);
- Dysgraphia.

While dyslexia is fairly common, its cause is still very much unknown. The NHS (National Health Service) states:

There are a number of different theories about the causes of dyslexia which all tend to agree that it is a genetic condition that changes how the brain deals with information, and that it is passed through families. (**www.nhs.uk**)

While the Dyslexia Association of Ireland explains that:

We do know that developmental dyslexia is inherited, only slightly more common in males than females and that one is born with it… Experts do agree that dyslexia describes differences in the way in which the brain processes information, and while there may be differences in the way in which the brain works, this does not imply any abnormality, disease or defect. (**www.dyslexia.ie**)

One thing we can say for certain is that around 10% of the population are affected by dyslexia, with 4% of the population severely affected. The issues can become apparent through spellings, short-term memory, visual processing, hand control, number work and reading. Dyslexia can also impact things like spatial awareness, interpersonal skills and timekeeping.

As those with dyslexia are often of average or above average intelligence, these issues can result in a great amount of frustration.

Why People with Dyslexia Are Successful in Business

If you're upset about your child having dyslexia, don't be! A 2003 study by the Tulip Financial Group found that a surprisingly high proportion of self-made millionaires are dyslexic, most likely because they've had to develop self-belief and dedication from an early age. Whatever the reason, Bill Gates and Sir Richard Branson are both highly successful dyslexics, and a strong link has been identified between dyslexia and entrepreneurship (Cass Business School, 2011).

Cass Business School have found that while just 1% of corporate managers have dyslexia, a massive 10% of entrepreneurs in the UK have the condition. The same research has found that those who start their own businesses in the UK are two times more likely to be dyslexic than the general population, while those in the US are three times more likely.

It's difficult to say for certain why the UK produces fewer entrepreneurs with dyslexia than the US – perhaps it comes down to failures in the education system. Certainly, the system in the UK is weaker when it comes to identifying dyslexia at a young age. Maybe if we got better at identifying dyslexia sooner, we'd be able to increase our number of dyslexic entrepreneurs just like the States have.

Girls and Boys

Although the condition was first identified over a hundred years ago, very little was known about the causes of dyslexia until around 40 years ago. There has been a lot of debate over whether or not dyslexia is more common in boys than girls. In research published in the JAMA (Journal of the American Medical Association), Dr Michael Rutter (King's College London) has suggested that boys are two times more likely to have dyslexia than girls (Rutter, 2004, 2007-2012). This study was based on data from over 10,000 children aged 7-15 who were given standard reading tests in Great Britain and New Zealand. Rutter points out that his results are more accurate than those of certain similar studies:

… the studies did not rely on children who were already known to have learning difficulties – a weakness that plagued some previous research…

That said, many people in the field of dyslexia maintain that the ration is roughly 50/50, so more research needs to be done on this subject. Early beliefs about the condition included one that suggested dyslexia was a "middle class disease". This belief came about because those in the middle class and above were more likely to afford to have their child tested for the condition, thus affecting the statistics. It's very easy to jump to the wrong conclusions when faced with incomplete data.

By now, we know that dyslexia is a neurological condition which affects the individual's ability to write, add, spell and read. Under the Equality Act 2010, the Disability Discrimination Act 1995, Education Act 1993 and Chronically Sick & Disabled Persons Act 1970, it is now an officially recognised disability. Fortunately, a lot more research is now being carried out into the causes of dyslexia, so there aren't so many wild assumptions floating about.

Medical circles now accept that the brain of a person with dyslexia is simply different to a brain of someone without the condition. The key to dealing with dyslexia lies in early identification as this will allow parents and carers to work towards a solution as quickly as possible.

Dyslexia and the Equality Act 2010

The Equality Act 2010 incorporates the majority of the Disability Act, which we'll discuss in Chapter Twenty-One: They Equality Act 2010. However, there are still plenty of employers out there who are unable to get the best out of their staff owing to a lack of understanding of how they can help.

Useful advice can be found in the information pack Dyslexia – An Employer's Code of Practice, released by the British Dyslexia Association. The pack provides advice and facts about the condition, and tips on how to make the workplace a friendlier, more inclusive environment. More information can be found on the British Dyslexia Association's website.

Adults with Dyslexia

In many cases, people with dyslexia are highly original and artistic. Despite their challenges, they tend to succeed thanks to their determination and diligence, and as a result are very good at working as part of a team. Some of the areas in which people with dyslexia may excel include…

- Architecture;
- IT;
- Electronics;
- Performance;
- Physics;
- Athletics;
- Mathematics;
- Engineering;
- Construction;
- Arts.

Identifying Dyslexia in Adults

There are lots of adults out there whose dyslexia has never been identified. Some will go their whole lives without diagnosis and may believe their difficulties come down to a failure on their part. This can cause major issues in the workplace when it comes to tasks like filling out paperwork because the individual will try to hide the problem rather than asking for assistance. Unsurprisingly, this can result in a lack of confidence, a failure to reach their employment ability and general damage to self esteem.

Others will notice their problems and seek help. A diagnosis of dyslexia can come as a relief as it will serve as an explanation for many difficulties, and an opportunity to improve their situation.

Do You Have Dyslexia?

If you have some of the difficulties in the following list, you may well have dyslexia. It is not necessary to have all of the symptoms for a diagnosis.

- Does your family have a history of dyslexia?
- Did you have difficulties at school?

When you're writing, do you…

- Struggle to take notes?
- Find it difficult to get started?
- Struggle with punctuation?
- Write messily?

In day-to-day life, do you…

- Find timesheets and paperwork difficult?
- Struggle to name the months of the year forwards and backwards?
- Have problems telling left from right?
- Find time management and making appointments on time difficult?
- Skip numbers or mix them up?
- Have difficulties repeating patterns backwards, e.g. 297, 792?
- Tend to dial wrong numbers on the phone?
- Accidentally rearrange numbers, e.g. 26, 62?
- Struggle with mental arithmetic?
- Find it difficult to tell the time?
- Have problems following directions and maps?
- Struggle with telephone directories and indexes?

When you're spelling, do you…

- Make lots of mistakes?
- Skip the endings of words?
- Mix up letters or skip them altogether?
- Find it more difficult on some days than others?

When you're reading, do you…

- Take longer than your peers?
- Often lose your place?

- Skip entire words?
- Read well, but struggle to process the text properly?
- Skip word endings?
- Have to re-read sections several times?

Dyslexia Hall of Fame

There are loads of accomplished, talented people out there who have dyslexia or related learning difficulties. How many of these athletes, designers, architects, artists, filmmakers, inventors, scientists, military heroes, musicians and vocalists did you know?

Athletes

- Rex Ryan (coach)
- Tim Tebow (NFL quarterback)
- Nolan Ryan (baseball pitcher)
- Duncan Goodhew (Olympic swimmer)
- Carl Lewis (Olympic track and field athlete)
- Muhammad Ali (World Heavyweight Champion Boxer)
- Diamond Dallas Page (world wrestling champion)
- Caitlyn Jenner (Olympic decathlon gold medalist)
- Pete Rose (baseball switch-hitter)
- Magic Johnson
- Jackie Stewart (race car driver)

Filmmakers

- Robert Benton
- Steven Spielberg
- Søren KraghJacobsen
- Walt Disney

Artists

- Leonardo da Vinci
- Sally Gardner (writer & illustrator)
- Ignacio Gomez (muralist)
- Tommy Hilfiger
- Henry Franks (product designer)
- Robert Toth
- Andy Warhol
- Jørn Utzon (Sydney Opera House architect)
- Ian Marley (contemporary artist)
- Georgina Chapman (fashion designer and actress)
- Bennett Strahan
- Pablo Picasso
- Christopher Lowell (interior designer)
- Chuck Close
- Ansel Adams (photographer)

Thinkers & Inventors

- Ann Bancroft (Arctic explorer)
- Steve Jobs
- Thomas Edison
- Albert Einstein
- John Britten (Motorcycle engineer)
- Dr. James Lovelock
- Archer Martin (Chemist & Nobel Laureate)
- Fred Epstein
- Matthew H. Schneps (Astrophysicist)

- Ky Michaelson (Rocketman)
- Dr. Peter Lovatt (Dancer & psychologist)
- Carol Greider (Molecular biologist & Nobel Prize winner)
- The Wright Brothers
- Pierre Curie (Physicist & Nobel Prize winner)
- Alexander Graham Bell

Singers & Musicians

- Cher
- Harry Belafonte
- Bob Weir (Guitarist, Grateful Dead)
- John Lennon
- Brad Little

Fighters

- Thomas Jonathan 'Stonewall' Jackson
- George Patton

How many of these physicians, surgeons, political leaders, writers and journalists did you know?

Politicians

- Winston Churchill
- Dan Malloy (Governor of Connecticut)
- Thomas Jefferson
- John F. Kennedy
- Gavin Newsom (Lieutenant Governor of California)
- George Washington
- Woodrow Wilson
- Nelson Rockerfeller

- Erna Solberg (Prime Minister of Norway)
- Andrew Jackson
- King Carl XVI Gustaf of Sweden

Surgeons & Doctors

- Harvey Cushing (Surgeon)
- Fred Epstein (Neurosurgeon)

Wordsmiths

- Scott Adams (Cartoonist, Dilbert)
- JF Lawton (Screenwriter, Pretty Woman, Under Seige and DOA: Dead or Alive)
- Stephen Cannell (Novelist and television writer)
- Larry Chambers
- George Bernard Shaw (Playwright, Pygmalion)
- Fannie Flagg (Author, Fried Green Tomatoes at the Whistle Stop Cafe)
- F. Scott Fitzgerald
- Jules Verne (Author, A Journey to the Center of the Earth, Twenty Thousand Leagues Under the Sea, and Around the World in Eighty Days)
- Eileen Simpson (Author, Reversals)
- Elizabeth Daniels Squire (Author of mystery novels)
- Lynda La Plante (Series writer, Prime Suspects)
- W.B. Yeats
- Bernie Taylor (Author, Biological Time)
- John Irving (Author, The World According to Garp)
- Patricia Polacco (Children's author and illustrator)
- Terry Goodkind (Author, The Sword of Truth)
- Richard Ford (Author, The Sportswriter and Rock Springs)
- Agatha Christie

- John Edmund Delezen (Author, Eye of the Tiger and Red Plateau)
- Dav Pilkey (Author and Illustrator, Captain Underpants)
- Jeanne Betancourt (Author, My Name is Brain Brian)
- Hans Christian Andersen

What Have We Learned?

- The phrase "Special Educational Needs" can be used to describe a great variety of different learning styles and difficulties.

- Until a special educational need is identified, it can be difficult to provide the individual with the support they need. The main issue is identifying what a child's specific needs are.

- Having dyslexia doesn't need to get in the way of life. There are a great number of very successful people out there with dyslexia and similar difficulties.

- The majority of children with special educational needs are able to stay in their original school with a little extra help.

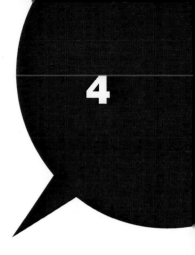

4

Dyscalculia

Dyscalculia isn't surrounded by the same degree of stigma as dyslexia is, but it's still very important that it's identified early to avoid damaging a child's self-esteem. While we don't know that much about the condition, it's estimated that around 5% of the population have it (Nfer-Nelson, Dyscalculia: Key Facts for Parents May 2002). A lot more research is now being carried out, so we can hope to learn more about dyscalculia over the next few years. It was originally studied by a Czech psychologist, Ladislav Kosc. Pronounced "dis-kal-kyoo-lee-uh", dyscalculia is a specific learning difficulty (SpLD) that affects mathematical ability.

The condition is characterised by an inability to perform tasks in arithmetic or maths. It can interfere with a student's ability to carry out even the simplest calculation or numerical fact, or to learn number facts such as the multiplication tables. A student may start answering a question correctly, but then switch to multiplying instead of adding as they've lost track of what they were meant to do. Sometimes, a child with this condition will seem to be getting on fine by answering questions verbally, but won't be able to say how they came to their answer. Dyscalculia, like dyslexia, often occurs as a result of a visual perceptual deficit. Put in simple terms, it's a severe difficulty with numbers. And just as there is no one way to describe all people with dyslexia, there is no one reason that someone might have dyscalculia.

Often, students with dyscalculia will struggle with basic counting tasks, or confuse small numbers with much larger ones. In many cases these struggles are made worse by a poor short-term memory or problems with sequencing and processing. It is essential to develop a pupil's skills in organising space, directional awareness, strategy, timekeeping, deduction and sequencing.

In the UK, dyscalculia is widely acknowledged as an SpLD. The British Dyslexia Association (BDA) believe that up to 60% of dyslexia may also struggle with dyscalculia. Just like dyslexia, there can be a great amount of variation in how dyscalculia will affect each individual.

According to the DfES (DfES, Guidance to support pupils with dyslexia and dyscalculia, 2001), dyscalculia can be described as…

[a] condition that affects the ability to acquire arithmetical skills. Learners may have difficulty understanding simple number concepts, lack an intuitive grasp of numbers and have problems learning number facts and procedures. Even if they produce a correct answer or use a correct method, they may do so mechanically and without confidence.

The earlier a student with dyscalculia receives appropriate assistance, the more likely they are to succeed.

What Have We Learned?

- Dyscalculia isn't surrounded by the same level of stigma as dyslexia, but it's still important that it's identified as soon as possible.

- If your child's issues aren't spotted and worked on at an early age, it can easily have a negative impact on their self esteem.

5

Testing, Multi-Sensory Teaching and Dyslexia

Your child doesn't need to be able to read or write to be tested. A few years back, you couldn't get your child assessed for dyslexia before the age of seven (or sometimes even later). However, there are now a range of tests available for children aged 5 ½ and above, and some that can be taken by children who are even younger still.

If you have reason to believe your child has special educational needs either because they don't seem to be reaching their potential or aren't able to keep up with their peers in classes, it may be a good idea to organise an assessment for dyslexia.

Assessments will identify not only your child's weaknesses, but their strengths too. They can also give a strong idea of how your child is performing in relation to their potential. This can be handy, as it saves you and your child the stress of under- or over-estimating their ability.

A test can last for anywhere between twenty minutes and four hours, and prices can range from £30 to £500. The longest and most detailed of these is the educational psychologist's assessment. Shorter tests are still useful, though, because they can easily and rapidly identify whether or not there is an issue, and sometimes the cause of that issue.

There are too many different assessments and tests out there for us to cover every last one in this book. Instead, we'll just discuss the ones that are most common and best known. Flip back to Chapter One: Knowing There's an Issue – Screening for a list of tests available.

Multi-Sensory Teaching

Multi-sensory means pretty much exactly what you'd expect it to mean: something that makes use of a number of different senses such as visual (seeing), kinaesthetic (feeling) and auditory (hearing). There's a massive range of educational games, computerised learning systems and successful teaching schemes out there including Hickey, Nessy, Units of Sound and Lexercise.

A number of different studies have found that methods that are multi-sensory and carefully planned are generally the best way to teach students with learning difficulties and help them to overcome their difficulties. As a bonus, as each difficulty is overcome, the pupil still gets to retain the extra skills learned in order to deal with dyslexia. When combined with perception and memory training and regular over-learning activities, a multi-sensory approach can help a pupil to participate fully and be successful in each area of the national curriculum.

The result is often a student with unique creative talents, exceptional ability in lateral thinking and a highly developed memory for sounds, faces and events.

How Can I Afford an Educational Psychologist?

Before you dive into expensive tests, it's a good idea to try out a free online assessment. If the test suggests there's an issue, then it's time to start looking into tests like the educational psychologist's report. There are private insurance companies out there that will fund assessments by chartered psychologists. Speak to your insurance company about their policies regarding this, and then ask your doctor for a referral.

Online Dyscalculia Test/Screening

There are a number of organisations out there with pretty good online dyscalculia assessments. Try checking out one of these sites:

- **www.dyscalculia.me.uk** – The Dyscalculia Centre;
- **www.educational-psychologist.co.uk** – Hit "Free Tests" in the menu. This website also has handy tests for reading and spelling;
- **www.quizilla.teennick.com** – Quizilla. Type "dyscalculia" into the search bar.

Online Dyslexia Test/Screening

There are a number of organisations out there with pretty good online dyslexia assessments. Try checking out one of these sites:

- **www.bdadyslexia.org** allows you to print out a test and work out your own score;
- **www.nessy.com/uk/** has screening tools for children aged 5-7, 8-10 and 11-16;
- **www.testdyslexia.com** is run by Ron Davis' Reading Research Council.

These tests can all be a good first step in identifying an issue.

Assess Learning Style Online

Everyone's learning style is a little different. We can learn more effectively if we understand and share our learning style. One great online test can be found at **www.educationplanner.org** (> students > self-assessments). It has a handy, simple to use tool for figuring out how you learn and what you can do to make the most of it. Another great site is Learning Pride, **www.ldpride.net**.

When it comes to creating an individual learning plan for yourself or your child, websites like these can be very useful. Generally, they'll show you what percentages visual, auditory and tactile learner you are. Depending on where you score highest, you can then work out what type of learning methods to emphasise.

A Broad Range of Study Aids

Nowadays, despite the misleading name, textbooks aren't necessarily just books. One of the main worries parents tend to have when their child with dyslexia starts school (especially secondary school) is the vast amount of textbooks they're expected to be able to read and the amount of homework they'll be given. However, the 'textbooks' your child will be studying from Key Stage 2 up to A Levels are mostly available in a range of formats, one of which should suit your child.

The varied formats will make it easier for your child to remember what they have learned, as there will be less emphasis on decoding written information. Available formats tend to include audiobooks (MP3, CD or memory stick) and films.

DVDs and Videos

When A Levels and GCSEs come on the scene, things tend to start getting more difficult for a student with dyslexia. This is slowly changing now that increasing amounts of work are being transferred onto DVD. Works like Shakespeare's Macbeth, Othello and Romeo and Juliet are all available on DVD now, which can come in very handy to students studying these texts.

Audiobooks

Calibre and Listening Books are the two main charities working to supply textbooks in different formats.

- Calibre supply over a thousand books to cover examinations and coursework. Audiobooks come on CDs or memory sticks in an easily playable MP3 format, and membership is free.

- Listening Books also have thousands of audiobooks falling in the categories of both education and leisure. Membership isn't free, but it is affordable and open to anyone. Many of their study guides can't be found anywhere else, and they cover the national curriculum from KS2 up until A Levels. Audiobooks can be ordered in the post, downloaded onto your computer or streamed directly from their website.

What Have We Learned?

- There are a great number of different tests and screenings available to identify whether or not your child has dyslexia.

- Once a special educational need has been identified, a multi-sensory teaching method will have to be arranged to support your child.

- Parents often find that they could tell their child had a problem from a very early age, often when they started at nursery or playschool.

- Whichever test you settle on, remember that it's best to have it carried out as early as possible.

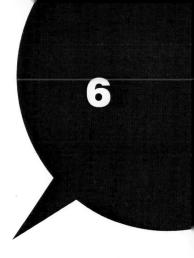

6

Dyspraxia

DCD, or Developmental Coordination Disorder, is a condition that affects your motor coordination. It affects around 5-10% of the population, with 2% of the population having severe difficulties. Other names for this developmental disorder include "motor learning difficulties", "clumsy child syndrome" and "perceptuo-motor dysfunction". In the United Kingdom this is more commonly known as dyspraxia.

We're yet to pin down the exact causes of dyspraxia, but many experts believe it comes down to an immaturity in neuron development in the central nervous system. As with dyscalculia and dyslexia, the impact this condition will have on someone's life varies to a great degree. Some individuals are only affected very slightly, while other cases can be much more severe.

The vast majority of individuals with dyspraxia are male. In The Medical Journal, the condition is described as "[a] serious impairment in the development of motor or movement coordination that can't be explained solely in terms of mental retardation or any other specific inherited or acquired neurological disorder". Although there are no set treatments for dyspraxia as yet, frequent occupational therapy and/or physiotherapy may prove helpful in improving a child's coordination and motor skills.

Unsurprisingly, the condition can lead on to real difficulties at school. Contemporary research suggests that more than 50% of children with dyslexia also exhibit symptoms of dyspraxia. In some cases, speech difficulties can occur and other developmental milestones are delayed. In many cases, individuals will also experience difficulties surrounding vision and movement, and will struggle with tasks such as catching a ball.

Recent studies have found that the difficulties experienced with dyspraxia does not end with childhood, and will often continue throughout the individual's life. If you are concerned about your child's development, you should consider talking to a health visitor, special needs coordinator at school (SENCO) or your own GP. If appropriate, they can refer your child for assessment with an educational psychologist, occupational therapist, speech therapist, physiotherapist or paediatrician.

You can find more information about the condition through the Dyspraxia Foundation.

While there is no real evidence to support the claims, some insist that taking fatty acid supplements like eye q and Efalex improves their child's condition.

Other conditions often associated with dyspraxia include dyscalculia, ADHD (attention deficit hyperactivity disorder), dysgraphia and dyslexia.

What Have We Learned?

- Occupational therapy and physiotherapy can be useful in improving coordination and motor skills, but there is no treatment proven to "cure" dyspraxia.

- What's most important is that your child still has the chance to have fun as much as any other child.

- There are lots of exercises you can do at home with your child that may be helpful, including trampettes, standing on one leg, balancing on things and coordination-based games.

7

Dysgraphia

t is not yet known what causes dysgraphia, but some researchers believe it comes down to damage to the motor system and/or a pre-existing language disorder. Pronounced "dis-graf-ia", dysgraphia is characterised as the inability to write properly regardless of the amount of attention and assistance the child is given. The main sign that someone is suffering from dysgraphia is that their handwriting is barely legible. This can be difficult to spot in children, however, as some will have messy handwriting due to lack of effort, while some may even write messily on purpose so teachers can't spot spelling mistakes!

Research is ongoing to try and identify the exact causes of the condition and how people with it can be helped. What we do know, however, is that it generally comes down to a physical issue with the action of writing. Sometimes, handwriting can be improved through regular practice. Some good handwriting books to check out include Why Johnny Can't Write, The Handwriting Rescue Kit (REM) and Unblocked! Dysgraphia Workbook (Inspired Idea).

Writing by people with dysgraphia can often appear distorted or "wrong", with inconsistencies in spacing and letter size. It's common for people with dyslexia and similar problems to write this way to try and hide their true challenges.

Will Exercise Help?

Exercises can prove beneficial in improving fine motor control in some cases, but many people with dysgraphia find problems persist despite practice. Occupational therapy can also be helpful in some cases.

Computer versus Handwriting

Computers allow you to focus on the work you're producing without getting tied up in aesthetics and the physical process of writing. For most students with dysgraphia, it becomes much easier to perform well when they're able to use a computer. It can be difficult to advocate allowing young children to use a computer because of the large amount of distractions and inappropriate material they may be exposed to, but in the case of children with dysgraphia the positive impact a computer can have often far outweighs the drawbacks.

This does not mean that it's not important for a child to continue practising their handwriting every day. Your child will not always have access to a computer and will need to manually write things down, and many studies have found that physically writing something down helps to commit its spelling to memory.

Sub-Types of Dysgraphia

A number of dysgraphia sub-types have been identified. Importantly, these are just broad classifications and there are many individual variations which can have an impact on prognosis and the types of assistance needed. In 1994, Deuel (Deuel, D. Developmental Dysgraphia 1995) suggested three sub-types into which dysgraphia could be divided.

1 Dyslexic Dysgraphia

In these cases, text that is written spontaneously will often be illegible, especially when it's complicated. While oral spelling is often poor, the copying and drawing of written text appears normal. Finger-tapping speed, which is used to measure fine motor speed, is also normal.

2 Spatial Dysgraphia

In these cases, both copied and spontaneous text is often illegible. Oral spelling is normal, but the drawing of individual letters is highly problematic. Finger-tapping speed is normal.

3 Motor Dysgraphia

In these cases, both copied and spontaneous text is often illegible. Oral spelling is normal, but the drawing of letters is often problematic. Finger-tapping speed is abnormal.

Signs of Dysgraphia

Checklist

The following signs are common indicators that someone might have dysgraphia. The individual does not need to display all of these indicators. If the problems listed below continue beyond the age where an average student has outgrown them, they may have dysgraphia and you should begin searching for advice.

☐ Very poor written text relative to language development;

☐ Writing is almost illegible;

☐ Writing in different directions, e.g. slanting to the left and then to the right;

☐ Letters of different sizes on the same line;

☐ Irregular and strange formation of letters;

☐ Taking a long time to copy from the board;

☐ Holding the pen too tightly or in a clenched fist;

☐ Watching hand very carefully while writing;

☐ Strange spelling;

☐ Difficulty spelling words, e.g. writing "brink" instead of drink;

☐ Problems with spelling words e.g. "stayshun" for station and "frot" for throat;

☐ Poor spelling;

☐ Holds pen very low down so fingers almost touch the paper;

☐ Does not follow margins;

☐ Very slow writing;

☐ Mixing up capital letters and lower case letters on the same line;

☐ Big and small spaces between the words;

☐ Mixture of print and cursive writing on the same line;

☐ Poor motor control.

Playing to Develop Skills

There are some great tools out there that many teachers and students with dysgraphia find helpful. These include…

- Pencil grips which help the student hold a pencil correctly;
- Pre-formed letter shapes children can trace with their fingers;
- Sloping Board Posture Pack to keep the page at an angle;
- Dexball which provides a "unique method to hold a pen";
- Software packages with word prediction and speech synthesis;
- Templates designed to hold paper at the right angle/position.

The best way to learn is to use multi-sensory methods during play. Some great examples include…

- Using salt/sand trays to practice letter formation (clean cat litter trays work great here!);
- Copying patterns and shapes;
- Writing on toys like Spirograph and Etch-a-Sketch;
- Following lines to find out which items are connected;
- Juggling;
- Swimming;
- Threading coloured beads;
- Colour by number;
- Tracing;
- Using coloured pens or chalk to practice letter formation on a white or blackboard.

Where Can I Get Help with Writing?

There are a number of groups out there who specialise in handwriting. For example, the concern of the Society for Italic Handwriting (SIC) is to promote good teaching and good handwriting. The group particularly hopes to support teachers at Key Stage 1 (KS1) who want to teach cursive writing from a child's first day of school onwards. They launched The Good Handwriting Initiative in 1997.

The main goal of the National Handwriting Association (NHA), previously called the Handwriting Interest Group, is to support children who have difficulties with handwriting and promote the improvement of handwriting-teaching in schools.

Which Softwares are Helpful?

There are a number of software packages out there that can be really useful for people with dysgraphia. They're especially helpful if the only thing stopping a student from doing their work is a physical issue. The programmes can take a while to get used to, but will save a lot of effort, irritation and time once you get there! These include...

- Word prediction;
- Spelling programmes;
- Mind maps;
- Report- and essay-writing programmes;
- Speech synthesis and more.

We'll talk more about software packages in Chapter Eight: Computers and Dyslexia/SpLDs.

Understanding That Practice Doesn't Always Make Perfect

Many people spend years trying to develop neat handwriting, and get nowhere. And in many cases, that's alright! At the end of the day, it comes down to what exactly is being tested. Are people looking for someone with perfectly neat handwriting, or are they looking for someone who can produce a good quality of work?

This is a very complex area, and until we know a lot more about it we won't be able to pin down the best way to help someone with dysgraphia.

What Have We Learned?

- Dysgraphia has only been recognised recently, and it's important that we don't stop at identifying it!
- More research needs to be carried out into the causes of, and solutions to, dysgraphia.
- People only started taking dyslexia seriously over 100 years after its recognition.

8

Computers and Dyslexia/SpLDs

There have been some massive leaps forward over the past decade in the field of technology. By now, there are too many packages of specialist software for people with different types of learning difficulties to discuss them all individually, so we'll just have to provide a brief overview.

Can Computers Help Students with Dyslexia?

Computers are quickly becoming a vital part of classroom teaching. There are plenty of programmes out there designed to be incorporated into a specialist-teaching scheme. While no computer package will ever truly be able to replace a good teacher, the right types of software package can certainly support and lighten the load of a busy teacher. Students with short-term memory issues can find assistance in committing information to long-term memory through instant feedback and programmes that echo letter names, and have fun while they do this.

Appropriate software can provide the carefully planned teaching, additional motivation, immediate reinforcement and feedback and over learning that many students need to learn successfully. They can help to build on vital skills, provide support for literacy and numeracy and provide structured learning to all students.

Computer Equipment – Hardware

The first three items listed are the bare minimum you'll require when working with computers. The other items are also very useful. The student's individual difficulty will decide what hardware is required.

- Computer (ideally a notebook, tablet, laptop or other portable device) These days, portable devices are the most popular computers because of their handy size. Most of these computers will incorporate sound cards (i.e. multimedia) and speakers, perfectly suiting them for specialist educational software. You'll be able to get one for as little as £299.

- Internet and email. Research and emails are made a whole lot easier with an Internet connection. If you can't get online at home, you should be able to do so for free in your local college, library or school.

- Printer (ideally one with a built-in scanner). There are loads of different types of printer out there. Many of these will have a built-in scanner so you won't have to buy two separate devices.

- Electronic gadgets. The dyslexic user can now choose from a wide range of electronic gadgets designed just for them. "iansyst" is just one of the many companies producing them.

- USB sticks. You can get an 8GB pen drive for about £5.00, and it's well worth this price as it'll allow you to download data and upload it on any other computer. The drives are easily portable too, about the size of a small pen or keyring.

Specialist Keyboards and Computers

- Keyboards designed for people with disabilities. Lowercase starter keyboards such as BigKeys are great for this. Here, any keys that aren't necessary for the student have been hidden or removed, making it a safe choice for very young children. BigKeys has an uncluttered, colourful layout in the "qwerty" style, and was designed for nursery and Key Stage 1 children. It's a great way to start a student typing until they're ready to move to a standard keyboard. The keys are very large and colour-coded to aid letter recognition: 'r' is red, 'b' is blue, vowels are yellow, etc. The keyboard is really easy to use – you don't need any special software, just plug it into your computer and start typing. Further information is available from KeyTools.

- Hands-free computers. These are more expensive than the standard computer, but can be worth it. The "virtual computer" is used in some offices and operating theatres. These special computers can be operated without a keyboard, mouse or touchscreen. Instead, you control them with hand movements in mid-air. These hand movements are picked up by cameras equipped with a pattern recognition software, so you can control the computer in the same way a mouse would. Their uses for those with disabilities are infinite.

- Touch screen computers (ideal for people with disabilities). Your touch screen computer will look just like any other monitor, but it can be worked by touching the screen with your finger. They can really come in handy when it comes to assessing children (aged three years and up) for early signs of specific learning difficulties.

How Can a Computer Help?

There are lots of different ways a computer can help students with learning difficulties…

- Problem-solving skills and sequential thinking can be improved by learning to use spreadsheets and databases;

- Students can receive reinforcement immediately;

- Students can receive essential over learning;

- Students get to listen, so ideas developed orally can be played with and easily altered;

- The student gets to work at their own pace;

- Almost every program incorporates spelling and reading;

- The colours and brightness on computer screens can be adjusted;

- Printouts and text on a screen are often easier to read than the student's own writing;

- Response is immediate;
- Most computers can now be programmed to "speak to you". This software could revolutionise foreign language learning. Programs with speech make learning truly multi-sensory;
- Students have the ability to make and self-correct mistakes in private;
- They can motivate people, especially children.

Computers in Examinations

The British Dyslexic Computer Committee

For many years, the British Dyslexic Computer Committee has been tasked with reviewing computer programs for people with dyslexia. They produce a series of booklets, which they update on a regular basis. You can find more information through the BDA.

Special Arrangements

It's stated by the Examinations Board Regulations for Special Arrangements that arrangements may be made to ensure that candidates with disabilities (such as SpLDs and dyslexia) can show their attainment despite their difficulties. Every examination board is different. However, special arrangements must not give a student an advantage over other candidates.

In order to find out exactly what each student may use, they must check in advance with the appropriate board. This has to be done a good while before the exam.

An educational psychologist has to have recommended any special arrangements used, and the psychologist's report needs to state exactly what special arrangements are necessary. That said, due to the limited number of educational psychologists available, additional training is available to some specialist teachers which will qualify them to arrange for things like extra time and readers.

Examples of special arrangements may include…

- Using a word processor (with the spell check turned off);
- Using speech recognition software during exams;
- Extra time;
- Use of typewriter.

Accessories

Recording Equipment

Micro Cassette Recorder (7-Adult)

By now, there are loads of these compact, tiny devices on the market, and they're all great for classroom note-taking. The Sony M800V is an excellent choice, ultra slim with good sound quality and extremely small compared to a normal tape recorder.

Digital Voice Recorder

These devices can be great for anyone over the age of 11. Several digital voice recorders are available, including the Olympus VN-1200 Digital Voice Recorder. This is an excellent recorder for note taking and dictation and can be linked directly to the computer. The device is small and simple to use, but it packs a powerful memory.

Portable Spell-Checkers and Dictionaries

PageMark Electronic Dictionary

This fantastic device is named "PageMark" after its super-thin design. You can slide it into any book you are reading, and it is always at hand to help you. Features include automatic spelling correction as well as over 145,000 phrases, definitions and words sourced from the Compact Oxford English Dictionary.

Franklin Collins English Dictionary with Thesaurus

Available from **www.mymemory.co.uk**.

Suitable for students aged 11 and up, this pocket-sized Collins UK dictionary features a thesaurus and phonetic spellchecker. Other features include an LCD screen, word games and ROM card slot. This is the perfect portable solution for students with dyslexia.

Pocket English Spell Checker

Spellex produce a great spelling corrector whose built-in databank gives students instant correction on their spelling. The device features Phonetic Spell Correction, which allows students to type the word as it sounds. It also boasts a Crossword Puzzle Solver and Matchmaker 6 educational games: Anagrams, Hangman, Jumble, User Anagrams, User Hangman and Word Builder. Other great features include adjustable contrast, a wordbank of over 110,000 words, and a "Confusables" function that tells students when a word might be confused with another by displaying the different spellings (their, there, they're).

The device is programmed with metric and currency converters and a calculator. When it isn't in use, it turns off automatically to extend battery life.

ReadingPen 2 – Oxford – UK

ReadingPen 2 incorporates the Oxford Dictionary. This is a nifty little tool to help your reading comprehension and fluency. ReadingPen is a life-saver tool for those who suffer from reading difficulties such as dyslexia. It's perfect for adults and children over the age of eight.

Personal Digital Assistants (PDAs)

These have one major advantage over any other small computer, in that you can edit and read your documents even when you're far away from your main device. There are two main operating systems: Windows Pocket PC2000 and the Palm operating systems. They are very useful for people with dyslexia and short-term memory difficulties. They generally have handy basic functions like creating "to-do" lists, editing and viewing data and setting appointment reminders. It's also helpful if you're able to find one that lets you sync up your files with the ones on your main computer.

Palm Zire 71 (11-Adult)

Palm is designed to help you get organised. Synchronise appointments and contacts with your PC ideas and notes on screen. More information is available from iansyst.

Smartphone Assistants

Most modern smartphones and similar devices will come with a digital personal assistant. The five main options are:

- Alexa;
- Google Assistant on Google Home;
- Siri;
- Google Assistant on a Smartphone;
- Cortana Invoke.

In a recent study[1], Stone Temple tested 4,952 queries on these five different options, and found that…

- Google Assistant still answers the most questions and has the highest percentage answered fully and correctly.

---

1   https://www.stonetemple.com/digital-personal-assistants-study/

- Cortana has the second highest percentage of questions answered fully and correctly.

- Alexa has made the biggest year-over-year gains, answering 2.7 times more questions than in [the previous year].

- Every competing personal assistant made significant progress in closing the gap with Google [compared to the previous year].

Pocket Word Processors

AlphaSmart Neo 2

Available from REM, this tool is perfect for anyone over the age of five. KAZ Typing Tutor included. A popular, inexpensive battery-powered word processor with easy, one-key transfer to PC for formatting. This amazing little keyboard can hold over 4,000 pages of single-spaced text and is a must-have for students and writers of all ages. As a bonus, it has fantastic battery life.

Software Packages

By now, there are probably thousands of helpful software packages out there. We're just going to discuss a handful of the more tried-and-tested options to support spelling, writing, planning, organisational, mathematical and reading skills.

Speech Recognition Software (SR or SRs)

Office XP now has voice recognition software built in. This software works by "talking" to your computer. The computer types up exactly what you say. Some of these software packages are now rated independently to be 97% accurate. Speech recognition software has really come on in leaps and bounds over the last couple of years. If you're buying a new computer, it's a good idea to check whether it's a "speech recognition ready" machine so that these options are open to you.

As you speak into the computer, your words will appear on the computer screen (already spelt correctly). This will help to improve the student's spelling, as they always see the words they're thinking of spelled correctly in front of them. The user will have to speak slowly and clearly, stressing the difference between words like "a", "an" and "and", but it's not necessary to speak like a robot!

The built-in softwares on programs like Microsoft Office are great, but it can be a good idea for students with dysgraphia and dyslexia to use separate, specialised voice recognition softwares.

Dragon NaturallySpeaking 13

This software is easy to use and allows students to create, alter and fix documents without the use of a keyboard. Price approximately £90. This is the world's best-selling speech recognition software, and definitely one of the best available for dyslexic students. Further information is available from Nuance.com.

Spreadsheets, Database and Word Processor

The most important piece of software for you to get your hands on is a word processor. Many of these will also feature grammar and spelling checkers. More and more, people with learning difficulties are discovering that the written world opens up to them when they use a word processor.

Probably the most widely used and trusted word processor is the Microsoft Office software, which is simple to use and has a good spellcheck and grammar checker. Many offices use this software. MS Office also comes with database, spreadsheets and speech recognition already incorporated. The majority of schools are happy for their students to complete some examinations and GCSE coursework on computers.

Reading and Spelling

Units of Sound Version 5 (9-Adult)

Suitable for Key Stage 2 to adult. As well as working on reading, this multisensory intervention program also works to develop spelling skills. The structured, cumulative program builds reading accuracy, vocabulary, sentence writing, spelling comprehension and listening skills. Units of Sound also includes a screening test to make sure the student is working at the correct level. You can access this program through Dyslexia Action.

Wordshark v.5

Wordshark is a powerful teaching tool for school and home. Wordshark combines the excitement of over 60 games with the task of learning to read and spell and is particularly good for students with SEN such as Dyslexia. Students of all different ages can benefit from its use, but it's used most successfully with students between the ages of five and fifteen.

GAMZ Player CD (7-Adult)

This program is based on the popular card games from GAMZ. It has many additional features and activities to support reading, phonics and spelling. More information is available through iansyst.

Nessy Programs

Nessy provides learning in a fun and multisensory way through videos, worksheets and games. Their goal is to help build confidence by teaching important reading, writing and spelling skills.

The company also has a variety of apps that teach phonics, syllable division, first words, letters and other helpful skills. Further information is available through **www.nessy.com**.

Speech Synthesis and Word Prediction

Speech synthesis and word prediction softwares "predict" what a student wants to say by guessing the word from its first few letters. In some of these, the computer searches its list for the most appropriate words, and suggests several of the most common words beginning with that letter or combination of letters. The user can then listen to the words out loud and decide which one is the word they're looking for.

Penfriend XP

This software is able to predict words before they are typed, saving time and effort. You can get further information from REM. A great help for those with dyslexia. It's also able to read text from documents and speak its suggestions. This successful product has been bought by every school in Northern Ireland as well as nearly 900 UK centres in colleges and libraries.

ClaroRead Plus

This is a word prediction program which turns paper and PDF files into editable, speaking Word documents through the ClaroView screen tinting program, Scan2Text (which uses OmniPage optical character recognition) and ScreenRuler, a strip-magnifying program. More information is available at **www.clarosoftware.com**.

Read&Write Literacy Software

Providing the ultimate support for dyslexic students and adults, this toolbar offers a variety of tools. It can correct words such as "there", "they're" and "their" where the sound of the word is correct but the context may be wrong. Difficulties with composing and reading written material can be overcome through a combination of phonetic spell checker, word predictions, dictionary and speech-feedback. The Texthelp company (and in particular their Read&Write literacy software) were honoured at the first DigitalAgenda "Impact Awards", winning the Education Category trophy in 2017. More information is available at **www.texthelp.com**.

Penfriend Portable

This product brings all of the great features provided by Penfriend XP to people on the move. You can use it on an unlimited number of different computers (only one at a time, though!) so it's perfect for carrying between sites and classrooms, and for taking home after school.

Grammar

Grammar Fitness Online Edition – Basic

This is a great online interactive grammar software with integrated progress-trackers. Students' scores may be monitored while they work with an easy-to-use tracking tool. High interest material engages students of all ages. It provides students with interactive grammar exercises to help them master difficult points in English grammar. The program is divided into levels, each of which teaches 50 grammar concepts through 1,000 questions.

After each question, an explanation of the correct answer is given whether the student's answer was right or wrong. The software was originally designed for students who need assistance with basic grammar, but it can also be used by adult students and English language learners. This program is available through **www.meritsoftware.com**.

Punctuation

Penfriend XP

A great help for those with dyslexia. Penfriend is able to correct a student's punctuation as they type, thanks to its smart punctuation function. More information is available at **www.penfriend.biz**.

Punctuate v2

Punctuate Plus lets you demonstrate punctuation in an entertaining manner, especially when used with an interactive whiteboard. This program is designed to motivate students to pick the best punctuation marks. Examples of punctuation, simple and detailed, are available to the student at all times. Dyslexic students can also benefit from help texts and a text-speech system guiding them towards the correct options.

It's easy to add your own new sentences to use within the program, and the speed tests promote skim-reading skills. This system allows you to make the most of one resource, as it works with all ages. The program is available through Xavier Educational Software.

Read&Write Literacy Software

See Read&Write under "Speech Synthesis and Word Prediction".

Maths

Key Stage Maths Invaders (All Ages)

Available from Amazon. Learn number skills by playing Space Invaders!

Numbershark v5

Available from **www.wordshark.co.uk**. This is one of the best maths packages, but it needs some adult supervision for programming. The structured learning program covers the four main mathematical functions: addition, subtraction, division and multiplication.

Angles, Time, Measurement, Shape & Space

This program is designed for KS3 students (aged 11-14 years). A variety of exciting maze-world allow children to practice and develop their maths skills by answering questions on numbers, time, etc.

Daydream Education: Maths Interactive Content Packs

These packs combine modern technology with great curriculum-based content to create a detailed but simple-to-use software package. The software contains easy to follow presentation screens to improve understanding, plus a wide variety of activities to reinforce learning and assess understanding.

Handwriting

Nelson Handwriting Series (Reception to KS2)

Nelson is a teaching tool for the whole class. It goes from Reception to KS2. Pupils can participate on the whiteboard by copying and tracing letters and patterns. Teachers are provided with a great motivating tool to teach core skills through animations and voice-overs for all letters and joins. The program also comes with printable worksheets that allow individual students to work on each letter and join in the classroom or at home.

HITT: The Handwriting Interactive Teaching Tool (Handwriting Without Tears)

This program is used by millions of students all over the world. It makes the mastery of handwriting a joyful experience for students and their teachers thanks to an easy-to-teach, easy-to-learn curriculum. The company functions under the belief that children who master handwriting are better, more creative writers. This program comes with pre-lined paper and is really easy to explain to students.

Study Skills

Studying has been made so much easier for students – with and without dyslexia – thanks to technology. There are so many great programs out there designed to help with organisation, reading, writing, note taking and time management.

Cogmed

This is a complete online system designed to improve working memory for students from pre-school right up until adulthood. Cogmed was originally developed in the USA and there is a complete supporting network with training and chances to try the program before signing up.

Mind-Mapping

Many students with dyslexia find it easier to work in a visual environment. This can make it easier to compose essays, take notes, revise projects and brainstorm. Mind-mapping softwares can make it easier to pin down ideas and arrange them into the correct order.

Inspiration v9

Inspiration is a fantastic tool for visual learning. It helps students to develop their ideas while planning and structuring their workflow. This software is perfect for students aged 7 and up. Students get to map their ideas out clearly in a neat spider diagram. Buy it from **www.inclusive.co.uk**.

Games

It's pretty common for parents to see games that aren't obviously educational as "just playing", but there's more to it than that! Many arcade-type games are effective in training the player's hand-eye coordination, and make learning far less painful than it might be in a classroom setting. Using letters and typed commands to make little men run around on a screen is way more engaging than typing out the alphabet over and over!

Speech Training

In some schools, children are now learning to speak properly with the help of computers. This is a project initially developed jointly by the Hereford and Worcester County Council and the Defence Research Agency. Thousands of words and graphics are available. Speech training aids display a word for the child to say and analyses the way in which the child says the word back.

It is then able to say whether or not they've said it right. Once the student manages to say the word properly, they're able to move onto a new word. Many teachers are amazed by the software's ability to "hear" the student's speech.

Software Agents

Some of the companies that sell these softwares include:

- Abbyy;
- Ai Squared;
- Claro Software;
- SEN Marketing;
- AVP;
- iansyst.

What Have We Learned?

- When it comes to education, computers can be really helpful.
- Specialist software has really improved lately and become far more affordable.
- Many people with dyslexia find that the written world really opens up to them when they use a computer.
- You can get software to help you learn a language, play the piano or even learn to cook.
- Over the last few years, in relative terms, they have become cheaper, making them more accessible for the average family.

Gifted Children

While readers many not necessarily agree that gifted children "belong" in this book (owing to the fact that they don't come under the definition of special educational needs), the educational system continues to fail to meet their needs, so it's important that information is made available elsewhere. Just because a child is gifted, it doesn't mean they shouldn't have the opportunity to be challenged and enriched as their peers are, and often that will take a bit of extra work on the teacher's part. As David Bell stated in 2004, primary schools are failing to meet the needs of their gifted pupils.

As with learning difficulties, giftedness can come in varying degrees. Some children will have gifts in specific areas like art, writing or maths, but for now we're going to focus on kids who are gifted overall.

The government's chief inspector for Education, David Bell, stated to the National Association for Able Children in Education in March 2004 that gifted children should be placed on a special needs register just like children with learning difficulties. If this were to happen, it'd be far easier to provide them with a suitable Individual Education Plan which would allow them to be monitored regularly and taught at a more appropriate level. For now, it seems that all LEAs are using different methods, some of which are simply better than others.

With so many schools failing to recognise their gifted pupils, it can be really difficult to get the needs of a gifted child supported. At present, we are yet to find a standardised way to identify gifted children in our schools. More than 30 years ago, Dr. Peter Congden noted the importance of identifying gifted children and set up the Gifted Children's Information Centre. The centre, along with a few other organisations, has been working hard to bring this fact to the attention of the government's advisors.

In 2002, the government finally listened to what Dr Congdon and agencies like his had to say, and the National Academy for Gifted and Talented Youth (NAGTY) was set up. In 2007, this was replaced by the Young Gifted and Talented (YG&T) programme. Sadly, these academies have both been closed. In a report published by Ofsted in November 2010, it was noted that most schools are failing to challenge these children.

As the report explains…

For more academically able pupils, inspection evidence shows that teaching and learning can be insuffiently challenging and poorly matched to their needs.

With the publication of this report, it's becoming more important than ever that teachers attempt to identify gifted children and provide them with the correct level of work and support they require to learn and grow.

Gifted Children's Information Centre

Dr Congdon founded the Gifted Children's Information Centre in 1978. Since its foundation, demand for books and articles on the subject of gifted children has grown and Dr Congdon has written various articles on dyslexic and gifted children, authored the new "Ant to Zip" series and addressed numerous international conferences on the subjects of giftedness and left-handedness. The main goal of the centre is to disseminate and circulate information about talented and gifted children.

Congdon's "Ant to Zip" series is a structured phonic programme designed to help teach all children, and especially those with dyslexia and other SpLDs, how to spell, write and read.

What Exactly Is Giftedness?

As with learning difficulties, giftedness can come in varying degrees.

Free basic IQ tests are provided by a number of online companies. Many people find it very useful to take part in these tests. One of the largest of these is Test the Nation, which is run by the BBC each year. You can access this test at **www.bbc.co.uk/testthenation**. Depending on the results received, you may decide to take a more formal test.

Other tests that may be of interest include those found at **www.free-iqtest.net** and **www.iqtest.com**.

Giftedness Checklist

These are just some of the signs that your child is talented or gifted. Keep in mind that they do not need to show all of these signs.

General Signs

- They don't seem suited to the standard curriculum;
- They have a wider vocabulary than most of their peers;
- They have a wide range of interests;
- They accomplish a range of things earlier than their peers;
- Good concentration;
- They find learning easy and remember things more quickly than their peers;
- They respond quickly to new ideas;
- Curiosity;
- They tend to ask very detailed questions;
- Deep engagement in tests;
- They can juggle more interests and hobbies than their peers;
- They tend to find adults easier to talk to than their own peers;
- Have strong opinions;
- Are often a group leader;
- Produce more elaborated answers;
- Are very imaginative;
- Will think of new ways of doing things;
- Will be the best one in their class;
- Are good at problem solving;
- Understand instructions well;

- Work well on their own with very limited intervention;
- Have a highly developed verbal aptitude;
- Have good general knowledge.

Maths

- Gifted children tend to have a high level of reasoning;
- Complete calculations with ease;
- Have a high level of visual spatial ability;
- Understand processes.

Literacy

- Many gifted children start reading before starting school;
- Are good at decoding words;
- Good at memorising things;
- Can comprehend complex printed passages;
- Read a book quickly.

Writing

- Gifted children tend to have highly developed ideas;
- Produce illegible handwriting (struggling to get words down as quickly as they want to).

Many gifted children show particular talent in,,,

- Music;
- Creative writing;
- Scientific thinking;
- Art.

IQ (Intelligent Quotient) Tests

If you suspect that your child might be gifted, it's most likely the best course of action to organise an idependent psychologist's test. During this test, your child will be asked to carry out a variety of different tasks, after which the psychologist will be able to provide you with a report of your child's strengths, weaknesses and IQ level. Once your results are ready, your child's school will be able to make an IEP (Individual Education Plan) for your child.

Mensa

Everyone has heard of Mensa, but do you know what "Mensa" actually means? Here's a clue: it's not an acronym! "Mensa" is latin for "table", the idea being that a round table allows everyone to sit around it as equals. The society has over 105,000 members all over the world.

Founded in England in 1946, Mensa is a society for very smart people with high IQs. All types of people are invited to join, provided their IQ is in the top 2% of the population. Mensa's UK branch, British Mensa has over 24,000 members, almost 1,000 of whom are under the age of 18.

Anyone is welcome to take a supervised intelligence test to find out if they're eligible to join Mensa. You may either take your test through Mensa, or provide them with evidence of a test by a qualified psychologist.

Mensa uses a range of different IQ tests on new applicants, including…

- Culture Fair. This test is used by British Mensa. A score of 132 places someone in the top 2%.
- Cattell B111. A score of 148 or higher places someone in the top 2%.

Whatever scale is used, all Mensans must be in the top 2% of the population.

Who Can Help Your Gifted Child?

There are many organisations out there offering support to gifted children and their parents, teachers and other groups. These include…

- Gifted Children's Information Centre;
- The Support Society for Children of High Intelligence;
- Pullen Publications (publishing books for able pupils);
- Mensa;
- National Association for the Gifted Child.

What Have We Learned?

- We owe a lot of gratitude to people like Dr Peter Congdon, who have worked tirelessly for over 25 years to promote an understanding of giftedness and dyslexia.

- Once their needs are identified, your child is far more likely to get the support they need.

- As the Internet grows, it's possible that increasing amounts of gifted children will be home-schooled.

- A start has been made, but it may still be some time before children are routinely screened for giftedness.

- It's very important for gifted children to have their talents recognised as early as possible.

10

ADD & ADHD – Attention Deficit Hyperactivity Disorder

It was once believed that this disorder was one that children would simply "grow out of", but we've since discovered that more than 30% of children continue experiencing symptoms into adulthood. As with the other conditions described in this book, ADHD comes with varying degrees of severity. The world has known about ADHD, or "attention deficit hyperactivity disorder", for quite some time. It's been about long enough for its name to have changed several times, from "hyperkinesias" (literally "super-active") to "hyperactivity", to "ADD" (attention deficit disorder) and finally settling (for now) on ADHD. It's a diagnosis most often given to children who move around constantly, have disruptive behaviour, perform poorly in school relative to their intelligence and struggle to concentrate. Interestingly, many children with ADHD also exhibit symptoms of dyspraxia and dyslexia.

Are There Different Types of ADHD?

There are believed to be three main subtypes of ADHD. These are…

- Predominantly hyperactive-impulsive;
- Combined type (this is the most common);
- Predominantly inattentive.

People with ADHD often seem to be incredibly impulsive and distractible, which can sometimes have pretty disastrous consequences. They tend to get bored after just a few minutes, and may struggle to focus on things. They often have difficulty with organisation and routine owing to their difficulty in paying attention for even the shortest amount of time.

It's believed that ADHD affects between 3% and 7% of school-age children. In severe cases, children with ADHD may even be expelled from school or end up getting in trouble with the police.

All children have the potential to be inattentive and over-excited every now and then, but kids with ADHD will be disruptive almost constantly. Although some research has suggested that the vast majority of individuals with the condition are male, it has also been suggested that this is because many girls will display the less immediately obvious "inattentive" form of the disorder. This is often simply read as the child being "dreamy" or "reserved", so they aren't diagnosed with the condition so readily.

Oppositional Defiant Disorder (ODD)

Often, children who have ADHD will often have ODD – oppositional defiant disorder. This is another defined by disruptive and inattentive behaviours, this time focused in the direction of figures of authority such as teachers and parents.

How Is ADHD Diagnosed?

For ADHD to be diagnosed, the symptoms generally need to…

- Have started by the child's seventh birthday;
- Be long-term (last more than six months);
- Cause real problems in at least two areas of their life, e.g. at home, work or school.

During an ADHD assessment, it's vital that everyone involved with the child's life has some input. Topics to cover should include…

- Family history;

- Toddler behaviours;
- Performance at pre-school;
- Home behaviour (it's common for this to be much better or much worse);
- Behaviour at school;
- Medical development;
- Behaviour as a baby (noisy, screams, difficulty sleeping, etc).

More information on ADHD can be found through the ADHD Foundation, at **www.adhdfoundation.org.uk**.

What Can I Do to Help My Child?

There are various things you can do to make things easier for yourself and your child. These include…

- Praising your child when they do the right thing;
- Rewarding their good behaviour;
- Avoiding overloading information by giving them one instruction at a time;
- Making sure you are directly looking at your child and making eye contact when you speak to them;
- Trying to ignore bad behaviour (when it's safe to do so).

Who Can I Go to for Help?

There are plenty of different people and methods capable of helping kids with ADHD. Examples include…

- Psychotherapists;
- Physiotherapists;
- Special support in class;
- Support groups for the children and their parents;
- Teacher training;
- Cognitive behavioural therapy (CBT).

Where Can I Get Help for My Child?

The Hyperactive Children's Support Group (HACSG) was founded by director Sally Bundy MBE and her late mother, Mrs Vicky Colquhoun. Their goal was to help people who had found themselves in a similar situation to their own. In 1980, the pair proposed the radical idea to the medical world that a link existed between ADHD and people whose diet lacked fatty acids.

Bundy and Colquhoun were the first people to confront medical experts and prove that they were more knowledgeable about the causes of childhood hyperactivity. They had no medical or scientific qualifications, but had noticed that children with ADD and ADHD tended to have other seemingly unrelated symptoms such as dry skin, allergies and excessive thirst.

The two women carried out a survey of over 200 children with conditions like ADD and found that their difficulties were most likely the result of biochemical imbalances. These imbalances were caused by a lack of essential fatty acids, or EFAs. Two such EFAs can be found in evening primrose oil, and it was found that the symptoms of children with ADD who took this oil were improved.

However, the medical community failed to take Bundy and Colquhoun's findings seriously. Almost 15 years passed before an American journal of clinical nutrition confirmed their proposal. In extensive research published since then, it's also been suggested that dyslexic children may also be helped by EFAs. These missing fatty acids are now available in a number of supplements, including eye q and Efalex.

EFA supplements are now available in liquid and tablet forms, and even in child-friendly 'chews'. Not content with the impact she's already had, Vicky Bundy has continued working to raise ADHD awareness, eventually being awarded an MBE for her work in 2005. You can find more information about her work and story on the HACSG website. The National Attention Deficit Disorder Information and Support Service (ADDISS) also has some great resources.

Do Artificial Colourings in Food Cause Behavioural Problems?

The link between children's bad behaviour and artificial food colourings has been debated for years, but research finally seems to support an end to the unnecessary, potentially harmful chemicals. In 1987, Professor Neil Ward of the University of Surrey worked with the HACSG on a study* of 357 children diagnosed with hyperactivity. Of those studied, 72% had adverse reactions to artificial food preservatives while a massive 87% reacted badly to artificial colourings.

*Hyperactive Children's Support Group > About Hyperactivity > Hospital Study

ADHD and Medication

If a medical professional deems it necessary after extensive testing to give your child medication, the least you should do is consider it. The medication most commonly prescribed to people with ADHD is Ritalin, also known as methylphenidate. The medication Adderall (also known as Dexedrine or Dextroamphetamine) was also recommended in the past, but has since been withdrawn by the National Institute for Clinical Excellence (NICE). A common concern is that medicating children with ADHD will cause them to become dependent on drugs. Ritalin in particular is villainised by certain groups, and is seen as extremely controversial. There doesn't seem to be much scientific support for this concern, however.

Importantly, medication should only be used to complement other forms of treatment, such as behaviour therapy or CBT, and should be reassessed on a regular basis. Whatever your initial position on medication, if nothing else works it may become a necessary "evil".

Is it ADHD?

The following may be indicators that an individual has ADHD, and all of these signs do not need to be present for someone to have the disorder. If the individual still has these issues beyond the time that their peers have grown out of them, it may suggest that advice should be sought and an ADHD diagnosis may be necessary.

Infants

- Frequently showing signs of distress;
- Difficulty sleeping;
- Constant and extreme thirst;
- Regular tantrums;
- Hitting their head;
- Rocking the cot;
- Screaming;
- Dry skin;
- Difficult to feed;
- Extreme restlessness.

Children

- Excessively impulsive and courageous;
- Taking lots of unnecessary risks;
- Lack of care around roads;
- Tends to have a lot of accidents;
- Overly comfortable with touching people and things;
- Talkative;
- Issues with eating and sleeping continue beyond infancy;
- Struggling to tie shoelaces;
- Messy handwriting;
- Poor self-esteem;
- Refusing to wait their turn, impatience;
- Sudden violence, such as grabbing and hitting;
- Lack of cooperation;
- Lack of obedience;
- Defiant;
- Inflexible personality;
- Demands must be met immediately;
- Problems with making friends;
- Difficulty with ball games;
- Difficulty dressing;
- Poor coordination;
- Allergies;
- Clumsy;
- Increased activity, always on the go;
- Erratic behaviour;

- May dash around;
- Do not stop to think.

In the classroom and other formal settings, the following issues may also arise:

- Limited attention span and poor concentration;
- Constant fidgeting;
- Tapping on desks, books, etc;
- Struggles with taking turns;
- Interrupting with inappropriate speech;
- Underperforming at school despite intelligence;
- Has a weak short-term memory;
- Blurts out answers to questions;
- Roams around classroom;
- Constantly moving feet, hands, etc;
- Sitting through lessons is almost impossible.

Adults

- Many childhood ADHD symptoms remain;
- Antisocial behaviour may lead to excessive consumption of alcohol and trouble with the police;
- Poor self-esteem may be distressing;
- Employment may be difficult because of relationship problems and poor memory.

What Have We Learned?

- Much of the discussion of ADHD in recent years has been negative, placing the blame on "lazy" parents and "naughty" children.

- A link between fatty acid deficiency and ADHD was discovered more than 25 years ago.

- We are yet to find a routine assessment for this deficiency.

11

Health Problems

There are any number of different medical reasons that a student might struggle at school. If you suspect your child may have a problem, this should be checked immediately. Perhaps the most obvious is if they are unable to respond, read or write properly as a result of not being able to hear or see properly. Your local opticians will be able to carry out a full eye test, whatever your child's age. Medical and hearing tests can be organised by your health visitor or GP. Some issues to watch out for include…

- Inadequate diet and overall ill health (e.g. as a result of a lack of vitamins);
- Glue ear (temporary deafness);
- Dyslexia and sensitivity to light (visual stress);
- Visual problems;
- Deafness.

There are lots of different health problems that might affect your child's academic performance.

Visual Stress (Light Sensitivity) and Dyslexia

Visual stress is not a symptom of dyslexia but 50% of those who have visual stress also happen to be dyslexic. People with visual stress may experience one or several of the following:[2]

- Blurred letters or words which go out of focus
- Letters which move or present with back to front appearance or shimmering or shaking
- Headaches from reading
- Words or letters which break into two and appear as double
- Find it easier to read large, widely spaced print, than small and crowded
- Difficulty with tracking across the page
- Upset by glare on the page or oversensitive to bright lights

In some cases any of these symptoms can significantly affect reading ability.

Specialists can screen for light sensitivity using a variety of tests and assessments, including…

- Cerium coloured overlays;
- Intuitive Colorimeter, Mears-Irlen' syndrome;
- Vision training (we'll discuss this in Chapter Nineteen: What Does an Orthoptist Do?);
- Dunlop Test (see above);
- Harris Filters;
- Visual stress syndrome (ViSS).

There are plenty of people out there who don't even know they suffer from light sensitivity. In some cases, children are only aware once the problem is corrected that not everyone sees fuzzy, moving letters on the page. These issues have been described under a number of different names including Intuitive Colorimeter, Irlen syndrome, visual stress syndrome, Scotopic sensitivity and Mears-Irlen syndrome, but all of these names are used to explain very similar difficulties.

---

2 British Dyslexia Association, Eyes and Dyslexia. https://www.bdadyslexia.org.uk/dyslexic/eyes-and-dyslexia

What Can I Do If My Child Has a Problem?

If you think your child might have visual stress syndrome, you can use coloured sheets called Cerium Overlays to carry out a quick and easy screening test. The Overlays are colourful translucent plastic sheets that you hold over a page of writing. You can get these sheets in different colours and if you find they help then you can organise a full test at the optometrists using the Intuitive Colorimeter or Harris Filters. When these are placed over the text, many students find that the words finally begin to sit still.

There are lots of handy, inconspicuous methods of using coloured overlays in everyday life. One product to keep an eye out for is "Reading Rulers (Duo)" from Crossbow.

Five per cent of schoolchildren aged between seven and eight years found that their reading speed on the "Rate of Reading Test[3]" was increased by over 25% through the use of coloured overlays.

Lucid ViSS – (Visual Stress Assessment Pack)

Visual stress can be easily identified using this assessment pack. You can purchase the complete Visual Stress Assessment Pack with test kit and overlays through Crossbow Education or GL Assessment.

If your child still struggles even when using the Coloured Overlays, a full assessment using the Intuitive Colorimeter may be necessary.

Cerium Overlays

The Dyslexia Shop sells the full Cerium Coloured Overlays Testing Kit and sets of Cerium A4 coloured overlays.

Harris Filters

Since 1996, Dr David Harris has been researching new ways to help children with dyslexia. Harris' range of special lenses that were originally developed to improve colour perception in the colour-blind are now making great strides with dyslexic students. He has developed award-winning Filter technology which has been found to achieve immediate and striking results.

So What Is This Award-Winning Filter Technology?

Harris' special lenses reduce or eliminate visual perceptual distortions, a condition that affects reading ability in almost 74% of dyslexia sufferers. Most people with dyslexia have nerve fibres that transmit vital information from the eyes to the brain ineffectively. This can impact their ability to control eye movements, keep their place in a line of text and understand what they're reading.

---

3   *Rate of Reading Test published by "ioo Marketing". Arnold Wilkins' book Reading Through Colour deals with this subject wonderfully.*

Of course, the Harris Filter can't actually "cure" dyslexia or make it disappear completely, but it does appear to be able to make reading easier and improve the overall performance of a dyslexic student. For information on where you can get your hands on tinted lenses, check out the Society for Coloured Lens Prescribers at **www.s4clp.org**.

Tinted Glasses and Coloured Overlays

Students often report problems with eyestrain, migraine, etc. One solution is to filter out the light that causes print distortions using coloured overlays. This should work in cases where black print on white paper appears to worsen the problems.

If your child has any of the following issues, they may benefit from wearing lenses or glasses while reading…

- Merging of letters into one blob;
- Letters dance on the page;
- Words swim around;
- Frequent blinking or rubbing of the eyes;
- Words look pale or faded;
- Words appear as a jumbled puzzle;
- Difficulties in reading and keeping their place;
- Words are fuzzy;
- Letters appear in the wrong order.

The Intuitive Colorimeter

Research has shown that if a child uses coloured overlays, their reading speed increases and they have fewer headaches. Professor Arnold Wilkins worked with the Medical Research Council to develop the Intuitive Colorimeter. This test identifies the exact colour which can help an individual student to read better by comparing up to 7,000 different tints. Special glasses can then be made for the children to use when writing or reading.

Plenty of newspapers have been talking about the wonderful success being achieved by scored of dyslexic students. Many national newspapers have been peppered with headlines like "A miracle cure" and "Experts cure childhood dyslexia using one simple trick!" This "miracle cure" is, of course, a prescription for tinted classes or vision training, which can improve a child's performance in class.

Obviously, this "miracle cure" won't actually help every single child with dyslexia. It has, however, helped a fair amount of children with this one particular problem, and is definitely worth a try.

Humble Beginnings[4]

Once considered to be a niche area of optometry and viewed with scepticism by some, the use of a colorimeter to prescribe precision tints to alleviate visual stress has become widespread, with more than 400 instruments in the UK and over 150 in many other countries in the world. Visual stress, or Meares Irlen syndrome as it is known, manifests as undesirable perceptual effects, which can be detrimental to reading and other visual tasks. The condition is thought to affect up to 5% of the population to a significant degree and 20% to a lesser extent, but using a precise tint or coloured overlay can alleviate the symptoms.

Vitamins and Health

In some cases, ill health can occur when a child doesn't have a well-balanced diet of minerals and vitamins. These days, we spend so much time in a rush that we can't stop ourselves from grabbing frozen and instant meals, but this can mean that our children don't get the vital vitamins they need to develop their mental capacities and grow at all. If your child has a healthy diet, there should be no need for pills as they should be able to get all of their minerals and vitamins from their food.

We'll talk about vitamins and supplements in greater detail in Chapter Twenty: Health and Nutrition.

Overall Ill Health

This title doesn't really need any further explanation. If you're concerned about your child for any reason, you can ask your doctor or health visitor for advice. If a child wants to access the school curriculum, they need to be fit and healthy.

Deafness in Children

Almost ten million people (around 35,000 of these children) in the UK have permanent hearing loss. Deafness is often associated with older people but many children are born deaf or profoundly deaf – others becomes so after an illness. A greater number still will experience temporary hearing issues during childhood.

---

4   *Extract from Optometry Today (Association of Optometrists).*
     https://www.aop.org.uk/ot/in-practice/practitioner-stories/2015/01/23/20-years-of-intuitive-colorimetry

Temporary deafness as a result of glue ear will be experienced by around one million children aged between zero and eight years old. This may develop into a condition called "acquired dyslexia" if it begins to affect the child's education. This does not have to be permanent.

Where Can I Get Help?

Action on Hearing Loss (previously known as the Royal National Institute for Deaf People or RNID) is the largest UK charity for deafness and represents the nine million people in the UK who are either hard of hearing or deaf. It campaigns in particular for integrated schooling (where applicable) and encourages greater public awareness of these problems. They also work to promote awareness of deafness in members of the public and the government, as well as campaigning for improved services and facilities.

Do Deaf Children Have to Attend a Special School?

A high amount of deaf children are able to stay in mainstream schooling. Many of these students receive the additional special education support they need within their own schools.

Checking Your Child's Hearing – The Newborn Hearing Screening Programme (NHSP)

The NHSP was started in 2005, and offers all new parents in the UK the option of having their infant's hearing screened during the first few weeks. If the test suggests there's a problem (or even if it doesn't) you can ask for further testing to be arranged by your health visitor.

Some schools even have a school nurse, so your child's hearing will be checked regularly once they start school.

Glue Ear (Temporary Deafness)

This is a very common childhood condition. The tube becomes obstructed by adenoids at the back of the nose so air cannot enter the middle ear and the cavity fills with fluid. The eardrum begins to appear dark in colour, and the fluid begins to thicken until it has a similar consistency to thick glue. Glue ear clears up very quickly, and the vast majority of children get it at some point.

In the rare event that the condition doesn't simply clear up by itself, general anaesthetic will be administered and a small hole made in the eardrum. A grommet, or tube, will be inserted and the adenoids will sometimes be removed. Adenoids generally disappear naturally at puberty, so children with glue ear won't need treatment after this.

In many cases, the only indicator that a child has this condition is deafness. This can cause their behaviour to deteriorate and their academic performance to suffer as a result. Hearing is generally restored to normal once the condition has been treated.

Can You Hear Me?

If your child has difficulty hearing things, it can cause real issues. Wax in the ear canal is the most common problem. Don't panic, though – there may well be an easy solution that will put things right almost instantly.

In most cases, wax will form into small beads, mix with dust and dead skin and fall out of the ear. Wax forms in all healthy ears, and only becomes an issue if the ear produces excessive amounts. Some people make abnormal amounts of wax and may have to have it removed by a doctor or nurse.

For most people, the ear's natural cleaning mechanism works perfectly and additional help from fingers and cotton buds is unnecessary.

NDCS: The National Deaf Children's Society

In 2015 41.1% of deaf young people achieved five GCSEs (including English and Maths) at grades A* to C, compared to 36.3% of deaf children in 2014. However, almost two thirds (58.9%) of deaf children are failing to achieve the government's expected benchmark of five GCSEs at grade A* – C (inc. English and Maths), compared to just 35.8% of other children with no identified special educational need.[5]

NDCS is a national charity that works with deaf young people and children. The ratio of children who are born deaf and those who become deaf in their early years is roughly 50:50.

Deaf & Blind

At present, there are around 23,000 children in the UK who are deaf and blind.

Organising a Medical Exam

If your school has concerns about your child's performance and ask for an Assessment of Educational Needs, a medical will be part of that assessment. This will take place in your own home, so you'll have every opportunity to discuss any concerns with the doctor in private.

---

5   National Deaf Children's Society, New GCSE figures show extensive attainment gap for deaf
     children. http://www.ndcs.org.uk/news/new_gcse_figures.html

Issues with Vision

Your local optometrists can test your child. Most parents visit their doctor and dentist regularly, yet many of them still do not appreciate the importance of taking their children to the optometrists (once referred to as opticians). Regular eye tests using new techniques may help to halt the trend of children with learning difficulties being dubbed "problem children", and would allow their difficulties to be identified much earlier on. By having regular check-ups (at least every two years), optometrists can pick up undetected visual problems. One of the most common causes of disability all over the world is visual problems. In the UK alone, around two million people – including 24,000 children – have sight issues.

It's been estimated by the Optical Information Council that around a fifth of all children may have undetected visual issues, and still 50% of parents with children aged eight or younger have never had their children's eyes tested. It's vital that a child has their eyes tested before they begin to fail at school, as it can be very difficult to restore self-esteem once it has been damaged.

In the UK, an eye test is available free for children aged 16 and below (and for individuals 19 and below if they're in full-time education) under the NHS.

Most children's eyes will be perfectly healthy, but some may experience difficulties if their eyes aren't able to focus properly. These issues can be sorted out very quickly by the provision of spectacles. However, if there is a more serious problem which the orthoptic feels needs further investigation, they can refer your child to the orthoptic department at your local hospital.

There's no need for your child to feel like the "odd one out" if they need glasses. In recent years, glasses have become much more fashionable, and it'll be easy for your child to find a pair they like.

Where Can I Get Help?

With the right help, blind children can perform as well as any other youngsters. If you need help with general sight loss, you might try contacting the RNIB (Royal National Institute for the Blind) who provide practical services aimed at helping people get on with their lives after diagnosis. The charity hopes to give the best possible start in life to children who are blind or partially sighted.

The RNIB are also working towards integrated schooling (where applicable) and a greater understanding and awareness of the issues faced by blind and partially-sighted people in the general public.

The Chronically Sick and Disabled Persons Act (1970)

You or your child might have rights under the Chronically Sick and Disabled Persons Act (1970) if you have sight or hearing loss or suffer from visual stress. If not, you'll more than likely have rights under the new Equality Act (we'll talk about this in Chapter Twenty-One: They Equality Act 2010). Both of these acts dictate that services must be provided by local authorities for people with disabilities. If the local authority refuses to provide a service, you have every right to complain.

Contact your local social services for further information. Your child will have to have their needs assessed correctly before you can receive any type of support through these acts. If your child is assessed as requiring a service, the authority has a duty to provide it (although they may charge for this service). An assessment can be arranged by the relevant GP or social worker. Try contacting your local Disability Service for more information.

If you have a complaint, your first port of call should be the council itself. Ask for a copy of their complaints procedures. If this doesn't get you the support you need, try requesting assistance from the local government ombudsman or Citizens Advice Bureau.

What Have We Learned?

- If your child suffers from an illness or medical condition, they may not be able to hear or see what's going on in class.

- This is especially important if they sit near the back of the class.

- If you want peace of mind, make sure that your child has received all of the necessary medical check ups.

12

Help is at Hand!

How Can I Get Help?

f you're worried that your child isn't reaching their full potential at school, your first port of call should be their teacher. It's common for parents to feel intimidated when trying to raise this subject, but this shouldn't be the case! The best time to meet with your child's teacher is generally after school, especially if you've called to let them know the topic of the discussion in advance. Often, parents will try to raise big issues like this in the morning, but this can be a bad move as the teacher is likely much busier than they look at this time of day. With thirty or more children, each of whom will need help finding pencils or taking off their coat, the teacher really has their hands full in the morning.

A good course of action is to call in after school, express your concern and suggest meeting up in a few days' time. This will give you both time to prepare for the discussion.

Taking Your First Steps

Make a point of keeping records of each interaction you have with the school. Whenever you talk to someone at the school about your child, whether by telephone or in person, write a quick summary of what was said. All this takes is a small, inexpensive diary so it's very simple. Try to get yourself in the habit right now, as you may well forget if you leave it too long! You'll learn later why this is so important.

Appointment #1

Before you leave to meet the teacher, compile a list that you can work through during the discussion. What are your main concerns?

- Are you worried about your child's reading?
- Are you worried that their progress is slower than that of their peers?
- Are you concerned that they don't have enough friends?
- Are they receiving any additional help?
- Worried about their spelling?

The list may go on.

If you're worried about your child's progress, chances are you're onto something. As their parent, you're bound to know them best! After the meeting, let the teacher know you'll keep an eye on the situation and contact them in a month to find out how things are going.

Skip forward one month in your diary and make a note. If you reach the one-month mark and there have been no significant improvements, it's time to make another appointment with the teacher.

Appointment #2

As with the first appointment, make yourself a list before you go. Work through this list with the teacher and determine whether either of you have seen any improvements. If the teacher believes progress is being made and would like more time, give them another month. Make another note in your diary so you don't forget.

Appointment #3

If another month passes and you still have concerns and feel like your child has not seen any significant improvement, make your third appointment. Write a letter detailing your concerns, making sure you keep a spare copy for your records. Address this letter to the school's Principal, but do also give a copy to your child's teacher.

When you meet with the teacher, exchange ideas and make sure you listen to their point of view. If you still aren't happy with what they say, explain that you've waited for improvement for over three months and are very concerned about the lack of progress your child has made. Explain (politely, but with authority) that you feel it would be appropriate to have the matter looked into officially.

When writing to the school or education authority, there are a few things you should always keep in mind:

- Always send your letter through the postal service.

- If you're sending a copy of the letter to someone else, you should put the letters "CC" at the bottom of the letter followed by the name of the person. If you don't have any way of copying the letter yourself, most post offices will do this for you for a small fee.

- When writing your letter, always work on the assumption that the reader knows nothing about your child. This will make things easier in the future if you need to get a solicitor involved.

- Make sure you always make copies for your own records and keep them safe.

- When replying to a letter from the education authority, be sure to see if they've included the letters CC and a name at the end of their letter. If so, you should copy your response to that person too.

- If you prefer, you can send your letter through Recorded Delivery. This costs a little more, but it means someone at the school will have to sign for it so you'll know when they've received it.

I'm sure you can see by now why it's so important that you keep a record of the outcome and date of each visit you make to the school. This will be very important in the identification and treatment of your child's educational need. You'll continue to need these notes later in the process.

Once you've sent your letters to the teacher and school principal, you've effectively asked for the first stage of assessment procedures to be initiated.

Your letter could go something like the one overleaf…

Your name,
Your address,
Your postcode.
Your telephone number.
26th June 2018.

Ms. J Doe,
Principal,
The School,
The Town,
Taunton,
TA4 5KB.

Dear Ms. Doe,

Re: Sarah Peters – D.O.B: 1st January 2009

As you know, I've been working with you since [DATE – check your diary!] on the subject of Sarah's ongoing difficulties at school.

I'm deeply concerned that she is not yet able to spell, write or read properly. As a result, she is being left behind and is growing increasingly isolated. She gets frustrated every evening when trying to complete her homework, and it's very upsetting for her. She now has very low self-esteem and no confidence in her own abilities.

I think that this has been allowed to go on for long enough. I believe that Sarah has dyslexia or a similar specific learning difficulty, and wish to refer her for a "Statutory Assessment" under page 42 of the 1989 Education Act (Code of Practice) so that she can finally get the support she needs.

It is my understanding that you have up to six weeks to indicate whether or not you will be carrying out this Statutory Assessment.

I look forward to your reply.

Yours sincerely,

[YOUR NAME]

CC Sarah's Teacher.

How Long Does a Statutory Assessment Take?

The time limit for testing procedures was set out in the 2001 Education Regulations. It was decided that the statutory assessment and statement process should take no more than 26 weeks.

In England and Wales, organisations such as the BDA and Network 81 have "befrienders" who will talk you through the Code of Practice and explain how to get what your child needs. They can also give you leaflets on how to get the best help possible for your child. The befrienders may even be able to attend meetings along with the parents, which can make the process less intimidating.

We'll describe the assessment in greater detail in Chapter Seventeen: Getting the Help Your Child Needs.

What Happens Now?

Once your letter is received, reports will be compiled from everyone who works with your child to identify the exact problems. The LEA will then examine paperwork from teachers, the education authority and the doctor and decide what help, if any, your child requires.

HESC (Health, Education and Social Care)

SENDIST (the Special Educational Needs and Disability Tribunal) ceased to exist as a standalone body on 3rd November 2010, and was instead turned into a new two-tier system of a "First Tier Tribunal" and "Upper Tribunal". Each of these consist of chambers that group together jurisdictions requiring similar skills or carrying out similar work. More information can be found through Her Majesty's Courts and Tribunals Service. Just go to **www.justice.gov**.

HESC First Tier Tribunal

Patents can appeal to the First Tier Tribunal if they are unable to reach an acreement with their LA (local authority) about their child's special educational need.

HESC Upper Tribunal

Instead of going to the High Court, parents can go to the Upper Tribunal if they aren't satisfied with the First Tier Tribunal's decision.

The Code of Practice in Scotland and Northern Ireland

The Codes of Practice in Northern Ireland and Scotland are slightly different from those used in England and Wales.

Scotland

In Scotland, new legislation was passed under the Additional Support for Learning (Scotland) Act 2004 which changed some of the 1984 Act. These changes included…

- "Additional Support Needs" replaced "Special Educational Needs";
- Children with a disability are no longer the only individuals eligible for Additional Support Needs;
- Requests can be made for all young people and kids with Additional Support Needs;
- Parents, young people and children's legal rights have been changed;
- New Mediation, Dispute Resolution and Tribunal Services were implemented;
- Coordinated Support Plans were instituted;
- Provision is no longer outlined in the Record of Needs.

Northern Ireland

In Northern Ireland, the Special Educational Needs and Disability (Northern Ireland) Order 2005 is used, which amended the Education (Northern Ireland) Order 1996.

Similar to the system in Wales and England, this states that the Education and Library Boards and Boards of Governors of mainstream schools are responsible for securing provision for children with special educational needs.

What Have We Learned?

- It's important that you talk to your child's teacher as soon as you realise there's an issue.

- Make sure your child's needs are identified and that any available support is put in place as early as possible.

- Give the teacher an appropriate amount of time, but begin formal procedures as quickly as possible if no progress is being made.

- Try not to be intimidated about the assessment procedures. There are plenty of people ready to help you at this time.

13

The Role of the Psychiatrist

by Dr. R. Eyre,
Consultant in Child and Adolescent Psychiatry

Introduction

There are Child and Adolescent Mental Health Services in each district. Referrals are accepted from all professionals working with children and often from parents themselves. They may also carry different service titles, e.g. Child Guidance, Child and Family Consultation, Child Psychiatry. Your local branch may be in a community-based clinic or a hospital setting. These now tend to be NHS resources, whereas they used to be run alongside education and social services.

The majority of children using these services will have emotional or behavioural difficulties that they and their families can see are causing them problems in their normal social or educational progress. Children will only have the same mental illnesses seen in the adult population in a small minority of cases. The Child and Adolescent Mental Health Services have a range of professionals who may be able to offer help, including psychiatrists, clinical psychologists, family therapists, community nurses, psychotherapists and specialist teachers. The Child Mental Health Services can be helpful in:

- Dealing with behaviour difficulties resulting from Specific Learning Difficulties;
- Diagnosing and addressing underlying Specific Learning Difficulties;
- Advising other professionals and agencies;
- Assessing overactivity and poor concentration.

In many cases, background factors will be causing stress that contributes to the problem a child is presenting. Examples might include family deaths, school difficulties, chronic physical illness and family break-up or relationship problems. Dyslexia is certainly one problem that may cause stress and distress in a child, leading to possible emotional and behaviour difficulties if it is not detected and appropriately managed in school. All staff working for your local Child and Adolescent Mental Health Services will have regular contact with the local authority, schools and nurseries.

Management Issues in Specific Learning Difficulties

When it comes to diagnosing specific learning difficulties, psychological testing is always necessary. This is generally carried out by an educational psychologist. The Child and Adolescent Mental Health Services' clinical psychologist may also contribute to the assessment in some cases.

After the child is diagnosed, the next step should always be to make sure that the specific areas of difficulty they have are fully understood by both parents and relevant professionals. Sometimes extra tuition from specialist teachers outside of school may be helpful, so long as there is good communication between school and tutor. Special needs provision will then be made by the Education Department for any extra teaching input deemed necessary, and it's also a good idea for a strong communication link to be established between the child's teachers and parents.

Sometimes the child and their family need ongoing support to help with these issues, and this is where Child and Adolescent Mental Health Services can continue to help after the diagnosis has been made. You can make a big difference to a child's low self-esteem or poor behaviour if you make sure the appropriate educational measures are being taken and the problem is being acknowledged.

Specific Learning Difficulties

A child has a specific learning difficulty when his or her performance on a certain learning task (reading, spelling, numerical skills) falls 28 months behind that which would be usual for that child's age and overall ability. Often, such children have good oral verbal abilities, so it can be confusing and upsetting for them not to be able to translate this ability into their reading, writing or spelling skills. As a general rule, the term "Specific Learning Difficulties" is favoured over "Dyslexia" by child psychiatrists.

Special learning difficulties can lead to many difficulties in the classroom setting. It is not difficult to see that children will often feel bad about their difficulty and may seek to avoid it by distracting behaviour away from the educational activity. They can also cause confusion with teachers, who may fail to see that the child has a specific problem and instead believe they are unmotivated or underachieving. They may be seen as misbehaving or disruptive in class when they avoid the work that is difficult.

Students with special learning difficulties can easily become nervous about going to school or develop a low self-esteem. Specific learning difficulties may be associated with other problems too. Research shows us that children with specific learning difficulties are more likely to develop later conduct disorders than children without those problems. They can easily move towards becoming a child with behavioural issues if the issue is not recognised early on.

This negative outcome is mostly to do with the problematic responses of the child and those around them to the learning difficulties rather than the learning difficulties themselves, so the movement towards behavioural issues isn't necessarily an inevitable progression.

Children with specific learning difficulties are also more prone to issues like poor concentration, over activity and difficulties with coordination than those children without learning difficulties.

14

Private Tuition and Choosing the Best School for You

No two children have exactly the same needs, so it's really difficult to tell you what type of school you should be looking at. The decision is completely up to you, but it's still a good idea to gain insight from as many teachers, parents and Education Authority advisors as you can. Most children just end up going to the school that's closest to them, but if you're going down the route of specialist schooling things can be a little more complicated because your options are more limited.

There are so many types of school out there. In some cases, just because one school might be really convenient, that won't mean it's the one your child should attend. It's really important that your child attends the best school for them. Try to visit every school in your area and find out what specialist provision each one has on offer.

Some school-types to look at include…

- State schools (mainstream schools);
- Specialist dyslexia schools;
- Specialist blind schools;
- Schools for deaf children;
- The independent sector.

You can find a list of all the schools in your area if you contact your LEA.

Independent Schools

Two main bodies deal with the independent sector. These are the ISC (Independent Schools Council) and CReSTeD.

The Independent Schools Council

The ISC hold a detailed list of almost every school in the independent sector. They represent around 1,300 private and independent schools all over the UK. This list features details of every school and notes any areas of expertise a school might have.

Schools on the ISC's list require parents to pay for their children's tuition. There is sometimes help available towards the school fees. Some LEAs will pay to send students to private schools, but as you may have guessed it can be pretty difficult to get this to happen. Some of these schools are day schools, while others allow students to board.

CReSTeD

CReSTeD is the Council for the Registration of Schools Teaching Dyslexic Pupils, and lists the schools that meet CReSTeD criteria. You can contact them to gain free access to this list.

Grants

Owing to the sheer number of applicants looking for funds from a relatively small pot, it can be really difficult to obtain a grant for dyslexia. There are, however, some great reference books that you can find in most libraries, and a few organisations out there who might be able to help you. One book to watch out for is The Guide to Educational Grants 2018-19 by Rachel Cain and Ian Pembridge published by DSC, £110. You should be able to request this book in your local library.

Mainstream (State) Schools

Most of the schools in this country are operated by LEAs and the government. These are generally "normal" mainstream schools. Children generally only move to specialist schools in "extreme" cases, where mainstream schools are unable to meet their individual needs.

If a child has special needs such as dyspraxia or dyslexia, it's common for them to stay in their original mainstream school. It's widely believed that this is the best option for both the child and their family. Some mainstream schools even have specialist units attached to cater for students with dyslexia, or will have specialists and therapists visit the school regularly.

The Portage Service

The National Portage Association or Portage Service is a home-visiting educational service for families and pre-school children with additional support needs. Talk to your health visitor for more information or check their website, **www.portage.org.uk**.

Their aim is to support the development of each child's communication, relationships and play to encourage fuller participation in their daily life with their family and outside the home.

Schools for Students with Dyslexia

Right now, there are only one or two schools that specialise in dyslexia in the state sector, while the remainder are all private. These are generally the best place to go if your child has severe dyslexia. Some are exclusively for pupils with dyslexia, while others just have dyslexia units attached.

Most of these schools will take pupils for a limited amount of times (generally around two years) before returning them to mainstream schooling. Children attending these schools are often happy there because they're on the same level as the students around them.

The Independent Schools Joint Council and the Council for the Registration of Schools have also approved specialist schools for SpLDs/dyslexia.

Schools for the Blind and Deaf

Lots of charities like the RNID and RNIB have their own specialist schools. They also provide guidance, training and support to state schools so that most kids can stay in their local schools.

PRU (Pupil Referral Units)

PRUs exist to provide education to children who are unable to attend mainstream schooling because of exclusion, illness or any other reason. Most students attend the PRU for a set amount of time before returning to mainstream schooling.

Education Centres

If your child struggles at school, private tuition can make a massive difference. Education centres have thousands of pounds worth of specialist teaching and testing equipment. Your child's school will be able to make an "approved absence" for education activities. Most schools are happy for students to take time out of their school day to attend these centres as, although they may miss some class, they'll be less tired at the end of the day and will be able to progress more rapidly as a result. The children are usually fine with this too! There are a good few private education centres all over the country that run from Monday to Friday, 9.00am to 5.00pm, and even on Saturday mornings. They generally take children in one-hour sessions.

Most students will come out of school for an hour once or twice per week to attend these education centres. This can be the best arrangement, as it may be too much for your child if they're expected to do extra work after school each day, alongside their usual homework.

Fees for these centres usually come up to around £30-50 per hour.

Other Options

Other schooling options include a wide variety of specialist schools that might focus on science, behaviour, dyspraxia, physical disabilities, dramma, art and any number of other things.

Checklist for Selecting a School

As you may be able to tell by now, picking the best school for your children won't always be easy! The checklists below will give you an idea of what you should be looking at. After all, not everyone fares best in their nearest school.

Specialist Teaching Unit – Staff

☐ Find out how many specialist staff the school employs.

☐ Are SpLD teachers provided in-house training by the school?

☐ How often does the school receive visits from other professionals like speech therapists and psychologists?

☐ Do dyslexic children have to take foreign languages? (Some schools allow children to withdraw from these lessons, so the student can have more special needs help.)

☐ Do teachers keep up to date with special needs courses?

☐ What qualifications do they have?

General

☐ Get yourself a copy of the school's prospectus.

☐ Ask if the school has a home/school contract.

☐ Ask to see a copy of the school's anti-bullying policy.

☐ Try to meet all teachers who will come into contact with your child, especially the special needs staff.

☐ What does the school do about discipline issues?

☐ Visit the school on a normal working day.

Specialist Equipment – General

☐ Will your child have access to special equipment like tape recorders, voice recognition software (VRS) and computers?

☐ Will your child be allowed to use things like computers, tablets, PDAs, palm-held organisers, notebooks or laptops for their coursework?

☐ Does the school use specialist software (recommended by the BDA)?

Specialist Teaching Unit – Students

If your child receives specialist tuition…

☐ How much tuition will they receive each week?

☐ Are the lessons provided one-to-one or in a group setting? How many students will be in a group?

☐ What qualifications does the tutor have? Remember, some schools use "helpers" who have no experience at all!

☐ In which cases would they contact a specialist (such as a psychologist) for specialist support?

☐ Are parents kept in the loop with regard to concerns and progress?

☐ How are details of the child's learning difficulties passed on to other non-specialist staff?

☐ How often do they monitor progress?

☐ When are these lessons held? (It is important that it is not during your child's favourite subject.)

☐ How is it arranged?

Private Tutoring

There are plenty of private tutors who work out of their own houses in the evenings. The best way to find a good one is to go by word of mouth, but make sure the tutor you go with is suitable! Many of these will be happy to tutor your child for around £15-£35 an hour. Some things to consider include…

☐ Are they qualified? Do they have an SpLD qualification?

☐ Do they have references? Check them!

☐ Make sure the tutor has certificates confirming police checks (from the Criminal Records Bureau or CRB) and that you ask to see them.

☐ Do they regularly update their knowledge with suitable courses?

During classes, does the tutor…

☐ Make use of multi-sensory methods like Alpha to Omega, Multi-Sensory World, Nessy, Hickey, etc?

☐ Use computer programs to back-up the child's learning and keep them entertained?

☐ Meet with the school when necessary?

☐ Test the pupil regularly?

☐ Give out regular progress reports, and do they charge extra for them?

☐ Give homework each week?

☐ Follow the recommendations from any psychologist's/school report?

☐ Feel qualified to undertake further assessments as necessary?

Resource Packs

You can get these from the BDA website. One great resource pack to get your hands on is the Dyslexia-Friendly Schools Pack which is updated regularly, free to download and available for primary and secondary schools. It has some wonderful tips, ideas and instructions on how to make your school a dyslexia-friendly place.

What Have We Learned?

- It's really important that the best school is found for your child.

- You may like to supplement your child's education with education centres or with private tutors.

- Visit all the schools in your area and see what specialist provision they can offer.

- Just because a school may be right by your house, that won't make it the best one for your child to attend.

- There are loads of private centres out there that can give your child extra tutoring every week.

- A bit of extra help can make a big difference.

15

Education is Compulsory – Not School

The law says that it is a parent's duty to cause their child to receive efficient full-time education suitable to their age, ability and aptitude, and to any special educational needs they may have, either by regular attendance at school or otherwise (Sylvia Jeffs 1996). It is education that is compulsory, not actually attending a school. Most children go to school in the UK.

But just because it's the norm, that doesn't mean it's compulsory. While it is difficult to ascertain exactly how many children do not go to school in the UK, figures of around 100,000 (approximately 1%) of compulsory education age children (2017[6]) are being home educated. Generally, it's referred to as

---

6   *Home Education in the UK, website: www.home-education.org.uk.*
     Wood, Mike. A Briefing on Home Education Regarding the House of Lords Bill H11 2017. 2nd ed.

"home education" or "education otherwise" if a child in the UK doesn't go to school. Owing to the general opinion of the state of education in mainstream schooling today, it's likely that the number of home educated children in the UK will continue increasing.

Children might not attend school for any number of different reasons. Examples of these might include…

- The parents are unwilling to let their children "go";
- Parents of gifted children may feel that their local school won't provide their child's education as well as they can;
- Students have been failed by some schools;
- Bullying can make mainstream schooling intolerable;
- Expulsion;
- Chronic illness;
- Religious reasons;
- Sometimes special dietary needs cannot be met at school;
- Some children refuse to go to school;
- Children with special needs need more attention than is available at some schools;
- Parents believe they can educate their children better than the state.

Contrary to popular belief you do not need:

- Anyone's permission to provide your child with an education;
- To tell the LEA yourself (some exceptions apply here);
- To stick to the national curriculum;
- To use the same timetables and rotas a school would;
- Lessons that are formal or school-type;

- To follow school hours;
- To follow a specific syllabus;
- To hold teaching qualifications;
- To justify your decision.

Education Otherwise is a leading organisation in helping and explaining people's rights to education at home. They have a wide range of books and booklets which explain your rights and duties and discuss the practicalities of dealing with educational authorities. For many years they've worked towards greater recognition of the practice.

In order to be home educated, a child must be de-registered in accordance with the Pupil's Registration Regulations if they're already registered with a school. Parents will have to write to their child's head teacher and explain that they have started teaching (home-educating) their child.

The procedure in mainstream schools is automatic, so the headteacher will notify the LEA as soon as the parents supply this written notification.

While things were tricky in the past, many LEAs are now fairly happy for children to be educated at home and will be able to provide excellent advice, tools and help.

Another great organisation to be in touch with is Home Education, who offer handy advice on education at home and dealing with legal issues.

What Have We Learned?

- While we generally think about schools when the topic of education comes up, there's a certain percentage of children who receive their education elsewhere.

- School is not compulsory, education is.

- At all times we must remember that it is the parent's choice and not the LEA's.

16

Career Options

Assessment Support at Employment Centres

All employment centres have been provided with a comprehensive description of dyslexia. There is a registered person known as the DEA (Disability Employment Adviser) at every job centre. They will have a great deal of experience and, more importantly, understanding of people with learning difficulties in the work situation. This is the person you need to talk to when you or another person with disabilities needs information about specialist vocational support.

Under the Equal Opportunities Act November 2010, Disability Discrimination Act 1995, Education Act 1993 and Chronically Sick and Disabled Persons Act 1970, dyslexia is registered as a disability.

Career Choices and Further Education

While decisions made at this stage in your child's life can affect their entire working future, thinking about career choices while still at school can be really daunting for a student. These days it's unusual to have a job for life and we have to continue to change and develop our skills over the years. The experiences we have in the workplace, in college and in school mean we spend our working lives frequently considering our career choices.

Job Centres

You can get loads of general advice on finding and choosing jobs and information about hundreds of jobs in your own area through your local jobcentre.

Next Step – Careers Advice for Over 19s

Next Step can give advice to adults over 19. Once known as careers offices, Next Step now hold offices in loads of different locations all over the country, such as libraries, health centres, community centres and job shops. The Next Step website is also very good and easy to use.

The careers advice provided by Next Step is available online, in "face-to-face" interviews and over the phone. Many people find them extremely helpful.

Helpful sections on the website include…

- Identifying your abilities and talents – finding out what you're good at;
- Career-planning information;
- Advice on building your CV (curriculum vitae);
- Information about free psychometric testing;
- Can advise you on interviews, what to expect, how to dress etc.;
- Has information on over 700 job roles such as, police workers, firefighters, teachers, care workers, gardeners, chefs etc.;
- Searches through many different courses.

Connexions – Careers Advice for Under 18s

Until recently, Connexions careers advisers were available to talk to UK students during their final two years in school. Sadly, these services now only run in the Tyne and Wear areas:

Connexions services in Tyne and Wear offer statutory careers information, advice and guidance services to 13-19 year olds (and up to age 25 for young people with special needs).

Following the Education Act 2011, from September 2012 individual schools and academies are responsible for making sure that their pupils get impartial careers information, advice and guidance.

Local authority Connexions services will continue to:

- Provide careers information, advice and guidance to young people who are in vulnerable groups such as teenage parents, young offenders, looked after children and care leavers

- Support young people with learning difficulties and/or disabilities as they move forward into further education, training or employment

- Help those young people who have left school but are not yet in education, employment or training

The services on offer from local Connexions delivery teams will be different in each area and each institution. For more information, speak to your Careers Teacher or Careers Co-ordinator in school.[7]

The new career service covering the rest of the UK is the National Careers Service, which was established on 1 April 2012.

National Careers Service

The National Careers Service promises to provide users with tips, guidance and information to help them make the right choices when it comes to training, work and learning. This includes support with:

- Building CVs;

- Finding and applying for positions;

- Finding training schemes and courses;

- Discovering volunteering opportunities that will teach you the skills you need;

- Learning about your career options;

- Creating a plan to help you reach your goals;

- Choosing training routes;

- Identifying key strengths and skills;

- Finding funding to support learning;

- Interview techniques;

- Understanding the job market.

---

7   https://www.connexions-tw.co.uk

The National Careers Service offer is available throughout England, with devolved responsibility for careers advice in Scotland, Wales and Northern Ireland. Their qualified careers advisers offer useful, impartial and confidential advice. The organisation also takes part in Adult Learners' Week and other national learning campaigns.

Skills Development Scotland, Careers Wales and Careers Service Northern Ireland are publicly funded careers services serving Scotland, Wales and Northern Ireland respectively, while the Isle of Man has its own dedicated careers service.

Psychometric Testing

This is sometimes arranged by schools and their careers advisers, as it can be of help to all students. It analyses the student's personal information and interests, then suggests career choices they may not have thought of. It involves comprehensive testing that can be carried out on a computer or in writing. These assessments can then create an objective reading of someone's personality and skills, and compare these against a database to match them with potential career choices. There are loads of different versions of this test out there, but they're all pretty similar to each other.

Are Psychometric Tests Worth It?

If your child chooses a career that does not suit them, they will soon become unhappy. It's really important that we find a job we like, when we end up spending about 25-33% of our lives there. So why not take the time to find a job that suits your personality? Nobody wants to hate their job! These tests are also available in some libraries, colleges and educational establishments, in some private companies and online.

Taking a psychometric test can help find you a career…

- That works for you;
- That makes you feel like you're making a real contribution;
- Which gives you job satisfaction.

Some of the more in-depth tests cost money, but you can also get some shorter ones for free. Some companies offer free online tests, usually have a very short introductory test and then you pay for a more in-depth one. Whichever you choose, it'll likely come up with some interesting facts and will be a worthwhile experience.

One free test worth looking at can be found at **www.psychometricadvantage.co.uk**.

Next Step online have free in-depth tests and you can start at a basic level and move on to a higher one.

Other tests can be found at **www.jobtestprep.co.uk/free-psychometric-test**.

These tests are really worth checking out!

The Adult Literacy Service

The Further Education Funding Council may be able to give additional funding to students with special educational needs. Your LEA also works with the Adult Literacy Service, who provide information and guidance to students with learning difficulties. Universities and colleges are responsible for making sure that all potential students are afforded equal opportunities.

What Have We Learned?

- Students at school are now given a fair amount of guidance and help.

- This ensures that the pupil has been given the option of different career choices available to them.

- Careers services generally begin helping pupils around the age of 13-14, and continue to guide them until they've left full-time education.

- You can access psychometric testing now through some universities, colleges, schools, careers offices and online for free. These are great tools for everyone, especially those with special needs.

17

Getting the Help Your Child Needs

by Dr. D. Cowell BSc. MPhil. PhD. Dip. Psych.

The 1996 Education Act is the most important law dealing with special needs. The Special Educational Needs Code of Practice explains it further. The Code of Practice gives practical guidance on how to identify and assess children with special educational needs. The 1996 act was modified by the Education Act 2005, and by the Apprenticeships, Skills, Children and Learning Act 2009.

Professional reports must take account of the Code of Practice and provide the required detailed information. This code must be taken into account by all Local Authority Schools, Local Education Authorities and early education provision who deal with children who have (or might have) special educational needs.

The Code must also be taken into account when Local Education Authorities are helped by health and social services.

The Code of Practice could be summarised as follows…

- ☐ The needs of all children with special educational needs should be met.

- ☐ A parent's views must always be taken into account.

- ☐ The child's wishes should be taken into account as much as possible.

- ☐ Children with special educational needs should receive a broad, well-balanced education which, as far as possible, is based on the national curriculum.

- ☐ Most children with special educational needs will have those needs met in ordinary schools.

Approximately 20% of children will have special educational needs of some kind at some time during their education. Children with special educational needs all have learning difficulties or disabilities that make it more difficult for them to learn than most other children of the same age. This is the legal definition for the term "Special Educational Needs".

According to the law, struggling in school because English isn't your first language does not count as a "learning difficulty." It is, however, very possible that students in this position may also be struggling because of an unidentified learning difficulty.

Here are some examples of special educational needs. Pupils may have difficulties with…

- All of their school work.

- Understanding what others are saying or expressing their own ideas.

- Sensory or physical issues.

- Being organised.

- A physical difficulty that makes adjusting to school and learning a struggle.

- Some kind of sensory difficulty, for example with hearing or eyesight.

- Behaving properly in school.

- Making friends and getting on well with adults.

- Some activities: reading, writing, number work, remembering information.

A small number of children – around 2% – will need a significant amount of support for the duration of their school years.

Schools are required to have their own special educational needs policy. The framework for action on these challenges is provided by the Special Educational Needs Code of Practice. The school is required to follow a graduated approach, meaning a step-by-step plan must be formulated to clarify or identify the exact type of difficulty a child is experiencing. It's also required that there is one person in charge of all matters surrounding special needs in each school. This person is generally referred to as the SENCO (Special Educational Needs Coordinator).

If the school starts to give support – such as extra time – to a child, their parents must be informed. In normal schools, this help is called School Action. This support is referred to as Early Years Action if it is provided in early education. The SENCO or the student's teacher will have to talk to the parent if advice from other specialists outside the school is required, as might be the case if the child isn't making sufficient progress. This kind of help is called Early Years Action Plus or, in the case of schools, School Action Plus. These external contacts include educational psychologists, speech and language therapists, specialist teachers and other help professionals.

As a parent, you can approach your child's teacher or the SENCO at any time. SENCOs should keep parents fully informed about the child's progress. Parental views will always be considered when decisions are being made, and the SENCO must always include the parents in discussions.

An Individual Education Plan (IEP) will normally be put in effect if the child requires School Action or School Action Plus. This document should provide details on…

- The nature of support being provided.
- The individual who will provide this support.
- Methods of assessment and how often these assessments will occur.
- What help you can give your child at home.
- What the targets for your child are.
- How often the child will receive help.

Depending on what area you live in, details of local parents' groups and voluntary organisations who might be able to help might be provided by a Parent Partnership Service.

In some cases, a child's difficulties might not be fully resolved through School Action or School Action Plus. These children will then be considered for a Statement of Special Educational Needs, as they have specialist, long-term requirements. This is a document that describes all of the special help your child requires along with all of their special educational needs. Children who require long-term special help normally have a statutory assessment. About 2% of these children will attend special units or schools.

A statutory assessment is only required if the school or early education setting cannot provide all the help that your child requires. This is a detailed investigation to find out the exact type of support a child needs.

A statutory assessment can be requested from the Local Education Authority by your child's early education setting or school. Similarly, you can ask the LEA yourself to carry out the statutory assessment. You will always be consulted before the LEA is contacted. If the LEA decides not to assess your child, you can appeal to the First Tribunal to ask them to change the LEA's decision. If the LEA carries out a statutory assessment, they will ask a number of professionals employed in the public sector to give their views on your child. Contacts the LEA may consult include…

☐ Your child's teacher or early education provider;

☐ A GP or other medical practitioner;

☐ Social services (who will only give advice if they know your child);

☐ An educational psychologist;

☐ Any other contact deemed appropriate by the LEA.

Parents can also send the LEA any private advice or opinions they have obtained. Sometimes the professionals may ask to see the child without the parents as children sometimes behave differently when parents are present.

If you contact the LEA yourself, you should always talk to the SENCO or class teacher first.

If the LEA decides that they do want to assess your child but you don't want the assessment to happen, you can contact the First Tribunal to have this decision changed.

During the statutory assessment, you have the right to be present at any medical test, interview or other assessment. As part of the assessment process, the LEA will send parents details of schools which are suitable for children with special educational needs.

As part of the statutory assessment, you should provide a written record of your views. These will be taken into account as part of the assessment by the LEA. After the statutory assessment, the LEA may decide to draw up a Statement of Special Educational Needs. You can request an explanation from the named LEA officer if there's anything in the statement you don't agree with. You can appeal the statement with the First Tribunal if you aren't happy with the explanation, referring to…

- Descriptions of your child's special educational needs (Part 2);
- The support your child should receive to meet those needs (Part 3);
- The name and genre of school suggested for your child by the LEA (Part 4).

The LEA must keep your child's progress under review and ensure that the statement continues to meet their special educational needs. Whether you opt for mainstream or special schooling, you have the right to say which Local Authority School you want your child to attend. You may wish your child to go to a school which is not run by an LEA. The LEA will have to go along with your decision, provided…

☐ You choose a school suited to your child's ability, special educational needs and age.

☐ The LEA's resources will be used efficiently in placing your child at that school.

☐ Your child's attendance will not hinder the education of other children already at the school.

Non-LEA schools might include independent schools and non-maintained special schools that might better meet the needs of your child. While the LEA is not legally obligated to pay for your child to attend a non-maintained or independent school if there's a state school that's equally suitable, they will consider your wishes carefully before reaching their final decision.

Local arrangements for resolving disagreements on this subject can be explained to you by the LEA. Before appealing to the First Tribunal, you should really talk to the LEA yourself to try and resolve the dispute. The First Tribunal only deals with a limited number of situations, as described above.

If your child has a Statement of Special Educational Needs, the Annual Review in Year 9 is particularly important in preparing for their move to further education, higher education and adult life. Depending on their abilities and requirements, they can stay at an ordinary or special school, or can move to a college of further education or into work-based training. A Transition Plan for your child's move to adult life should be discussed during this review. Your child's statement must be reviewed at least once every year, but this can happen more often if the LEA deems it necessary.

Education doesn't end at the age of 16 for young people with special educational needs. Your child probably won't keep their statement if they leave school to seek further education. Their college will, however, be able to provide appropriate support and continue to monitor their progress.

If you have a complaint that can't be dealt with by the First Tribunal, the local government Ombudsman may be able to help you. For example, you might contact them if required time limits aren't being met by the LEA.

A guide for parents and carers – called Special Educational Needs – is produced by the Department for Education (DfE). One important point made by this publication is that it can be a good idea for parents to talk to an independent body familiar with special educational needs. For example, you could refer to your own psychologist or medical practitioner. They will usually have substantial experience in either the Health Service or Local Education Authorities, or both. One reason for obtaining independent advice is that the person you see may be able to be more objective than someone who is, for example, employed by the LEA with whom you are negotiating.

The guide also explains that you can find support through national and local charities and voluntary organisations, as well as the local Parent Partnership Service. Families who have private health insurance can sometimes obtain the help of a private practitioner through the insurance scheme.

This will provide you with the advantage of choosing your own support system. A lot of private practitioners have a great amount of experience in special educational needs and its specialised areas. A further advantage is that the private practitioner would be available to you if the child moves to a new school, or if you move to a new area.

The professional body over most private practitioners will have set down a code of practice which your practitioner must follow. It's also likely that they'll have their own professional indemnity insurance.

Two names and addresses are particularly important for parents to know about. SENDIST[8], the Special Educational Needs Tribunal, provide a great booklet which you can access through the SEN Tribunal or LEA. Meanwhile, a booklet with information on the local government Ombudsman is available through the Ombudsman's office or LEA.

If your child moves schools or you move to a new area, this will often mean a complete change in the professional personnel with whom your child is involved within the National Health Service or LEA.

If you access support from a private practitioner, you'll have to take their advice into account as part of the LEA assessment. This is explained further in the Special Educational Needs booklet.

Initial appeals by parents against the proposed decisions of Local Education Authorities will go by the First Tribunal. As explained earlier in the book, the First Tribunal and Upper Tribunal now form a two-tier structure. These changes are likely to require parents to seek, and pay for, advice from legally-qualified individuals (i.e. solicitors and barristers), rather than educational psychologists. This is a result of the appeals process focussing more on the ideas of definition and precedent.

If you aren't happy with your result in the First Tribunal, you can contact the Upper Tribunal to lodge an appeal.

An important point for parents to bear in mind, is that no longer is the Local Education Authority required to pay for the best possible educational placement for a pupil regardless of cost. They removed this obligation more than 20 years ago. It's now expected that a Tribunal will take costs into account instead of simply the educational benefits.

Whatever your result, educational psychologists will continue to play an important part in the process. They'll be responsible for things like explaining the complex problems around clinical and statistical prediction; understanding the possibilities of common and unusual teaching and remedial techniques; knowing the limitations and opportunities posed by standardised tests, and carrying out detailed diagnoses over long stretches of time.

---

8   These arrangements came into effect on the 3rd November 2010.

Many psychologists believe that these roles can only be carried out by highly experienced individuals who specialise in the exact subject of the appealed case. This means that it can be very difficult (and expensive) to find a suitably qualified psychologist.

Many parents feel that educational psychologists working for the local authority are being paid to work against them. But many of these psychologists have been found to resist pressure to modify or alter their views, as their professional role's terms require them to be impartial.

The hierarchical nature of the LEA can often cause problems for parents. In some cases, the LEA will not send the educational psychologist who has been supporting and advising a family to appear before the Upper or First Tier Tribunal. Instead, they'll send an "Education Officer" or a Senior or Principal Educational Psychologist, saying this person has more experience with the issues involved in the case.

In most families, time, energy and money are limited. Parents really should think twice before choosing to embark on an appeal process that is likely to turn out exhausting, frustrating and painfully drawn-out. A further word of caution is due with regard to the reasons for the appeal. Many courses of "treatment" or educational procedures are based on remarkably little evidence and cost many thousands of pounds every month, for perhaps years.

Always keep in mind the potential dangers to family bonds that can come hand in hand with cases that last months or years, such as siblings who feel that this focus on one family member has caused them to be ignored.

It's not uncommon for families to fight for a course of action without realising how little evidence supports that type of treatment. Three examples of such "lost causes" that have happened over the years include…

- The dubious idea that children would make better progress in literacy if they were given "counselling". This was based on the idea of improving their self-esteem.

- For around 5 years, one company offered programmes that claimed to cure a number of conditions like dyslexia, ADD, ADHD and dyspraxia. The programme was based on a set of exercised said to be based on those prescribed to "spacemen" who supposedly experienced symptoms similar to those of dyslexia after spending time with no gravity.

- The last example was based on "recapitulation", a nineteenth century theory. This aimed to reactivate the walking and balance reflexes of our reptilian and ape-like ancestors, and involved exercises that lasted for several hours every day.

The vendors of these schemes not only managed to obtain worldwide publicity for their claims, but they were able to recruit well-meaning and sincere members of the public to work for them. However, in general the only "evidence" available was that issued by the company selling the programme. No scientific evidence was available to support these cases, just as none is available to support some of the options available today.

Inspiring stories about people who made amazing progress after every other method had failed them were used invariably to answer enquiries about the value for these programmes.

Northern Ireland and Scotland

The Code of Practice used in Northern Ireland and Scotland is different to the one used in England and Wales. We discussed this Code of Practice in Chapter Twelve: Help is at Hand! .

18

Legal Advice

I n some cases, no matter how hard a parent tries to get their child the help they need, things still refuse to fall into place. These parents may decide to get legal help, having exhausted all of their other options.

Ms Pamela Phelps, a former pupil aged 26 at the time of the court case, was awarded over £46,000 when she sued the London Borough of Hillingdon because they failed to have her dyslexia diagnosed.

In a similar case, Stockport County Court awarded Mr Robin Johnson compensation of over £50,000 plus costs when he revealed that his teachers had failed to detect his dyslexia for almost ten years. With these type of monies, being paid out by local authorities, it is really in their interests to sort problems out before they intensify to this level. Johnson explained that he was let down during his early school days, and as a result was not able to reach his full potential at school.

When looking for a company, please ensure the legal firms are registered with the Education Law Association. These associations are regulated by the Law Society. Legal advice is offered by a number of specialist firms who help people who have had problems with their colleges and LEAs for any reason.

All aspects of education law can generally by these companies, including…

- Details of statementing and assessments;
- Enforcing a statement;
- Tribunals dealing with special educational needs;
- Working with schools that want to cut down your child's therapy and teaching time;
- Information about provision from your school or LEA;
- What to do if your child is excluded from school;
- Bullying;
- Students who are failed by their schools;
- Home tuition;
- School refusals;
- Independent school placements;
- Finding suitable experts for diagnosis of your child's needs;
- Admission to schools you have chosen;
- Special educational needs;
- Statementing procedures.

19

What Does an Orthoptist Do?

by Christine Robinson (Mrs) DBO, SRO.
Senior Orthoptist, Great Western Hospital, Swindon

The tests carried out by the orthoptist help to analyse whether there are any contributory visual problems associated with the learning difficulties a child experiences. They are specially trained therapists who, among other things, assess vision for close work and distance and binocular function (how well the two eyes work together). It can sometimes be necessary for children with specific learning difficulties to obtain a referral for a Dunlop Test with the orthoptist. In these cases, the orthoptist is well qualified to carry out the test. They do not promise a miraculous cure if treatment is undertaken, but it may improve the visual information processing which can cause great problems for these children.

The Dunlop Test is one small part of your child's orthoptic assessment. There are some orthoptists who specialise in the assessment of children with dyslexia and related conditions. In most cases, specialised teaching will still be necessary for these children.

What Will the Testing Involve?

As a general rule, your orthoptist will want details of any past treatments for eye problems in order to build a full history. Testing will then consist things like…

- Testing to deal with "cross eyes", caused by squinting;
- Testing convergence: the ability of the eyes to look in at a close target;
- Testing 3D (stereoscopic) vision;
- Testing whether there is a well established reference eye (The Dunlop Test);
- Testing with the Dyslexia Research Trust's blue and yellow filters (if appropriate);
- Assessment with a selection of intuitive coloured overlays, if considered appropriate. If the child thinks one of the overlays helps, a rate of reading test is undertaken both with and without the choice filter;
- Tests on the reserves of muscle ability present to maintain comfortable use of both eyes together;
- Assessing the ability of both eyes to focus clearly on print at a near point, i.e. accommodation;
- Checking of eye movements and ability to scan and pursue a moving target.

Once the tests are completed, your orthoptist will be able to discuss the findings with you.

Will Treatment Be Needed?

If the intuitive coloured overlays are helpful, the child can be referred to an optometrist with a "colorimeter" – this is a machine to determine the exact colour to be dispensed in tinted glasses. These glasses are great because they'll come in handy for both reading and writing.

If there is no reference eye and the child is over seven, special glasses with one lens frosted over may be prescribed for all reading, writing and number work. If your child already has a fixed reference eye then it is unlikely that frosted glass will be needed. In cases where the child's vision is reduced, they'll require an appointment with an ophthalmologist (specialist eye doctor) or optician to find out if glasses are required and if the eyes are healthy.

These treatments are in no way "self-help", and the orthoptist will need to monitor your child's progress carefully.

In some cases, eye exercises can help children with dyslexia to use both of their eyes together at a near point more accurately. Often it's only when they begin to receive treatment that children will actually admit that letters and words have been going fuzzy or dancing around – if nobody's shown them how these things are meant to look, how are they to know that not everyone sees those things?

Tinted glasses can be offered on loan for either colour if the orthoptist decides on a Dyslexia Research Trust filter.

Treatment Goals

☐ Helping your child to develop a reference eye;

☐ Developing smoother eye movements during pursuit and scan;

☐ To have good muscle reserves (fusional ability);

☐ To have a good ability to look in to a near point with both eyes together, and maintain a clear picture (convergence and accommodation).

Optometric Evaluation

by Keith Holland, BSc, FBCO, DCLP.

If a child is to absorb information, stay interested and concentrate on written words, certain capabilities need to have developed within their visual system. Their eyes need to be able to jump back and down to the beginning of the next line and move comfortably and smoothly along a line of print repeatedly for extended periods.

When it comes to copying from the blackboard, the student will also have to be able to adjust the focus of their eyes between a distant board and nearby page quite rapidly.

Learning to Read

Some young people fail to develop these skills and as a result their reading and writing ability is often lower than expected. An action needs to be learned if you want your child to be able to move their eyes in a way that allows them to read efficiently.

Children whose vision systems are improperly developed are often seen to be ill-coordinated and ungraceful, which can impact other skills like gymnastics and even catching a ball.

How Do I Get an Appointment with the Orthoptist?

Some orthoptists are happy to see private patients and in this instance a referral letter from your GP is not always essential. If you want an NHS referral, you'll need a letter of introduction from the school nurse or GP. Not all orthoptic departments are able to undertake every test, so you'll need to look up the availability of the appropriate tests in your area first.

The Dunlop Test

Much research has been conducted in this country by Dr J. Stein, a physiologist, and Mrs S. Fowler, an orthoptist (Royal Berkshire Hospital, Reading). Developed in Australia in 1971, the Dunlop Test was designed by an orthoptist called Mrs. P. Dunlop. It is a two-eyed test – both eyes are open – and we learn whether a reference or lead eye is established.

The Dunlop Test involves looking at pictures through a special machine, so that the orthoptist can work out which eye is responsible for sending messages (pictures) to the brain's language centre so that they can be translated into words.

Reference and lead eyes are not to be confused with the dominant eye, which is tested simply by holding a kaleidoscope or tube up to one eye. The dominant eye will remain open, while the other will usually close automatically.

How Long Will This Treatment Take?

If treatment is suggested, it is certainly worth a try as there is nothing to lose and it may prove to be extremely beneficial. If treatment is recommended, it might last for anywhere between a month (for eye exercises) and a year (for frosted glasses).

If your child has received treatment for a full year without developing a reference eye, the orthoptist will stop treatment.

Subconscious or Deliberate?

If the brain has to "use up" concentration and energy in order to simply move the eyes along a line of print, then there is less likelihood that the contents of the text will have any meaning, that they will be remembered or that the words which are coming next are anticipated. It's vital that the basic eye movements associated with reading can be carried out without conscious effort or thought. The act of reading needs to become subconscious.

Visual Skills Are Trainable

Behaviour optometrists operate on the basis that visual skills are learned and therefore trainable. Behaviour optometry is now practiced by certain state registered and fully qualified optometrists. Behavioural optometrists use activities and training to improve the efficiency of the whole visual system.

We shouldn't regard vision as an individual, distinct function as it's considered to be an inseparable part if the whole human system. What this means is that our environment and our actions can have an effect on how our visual system works, and that our visual system can have an effect on our behaviour.

Who Can Benefit?

Optometric vision training is individually programmed to the specific needs of each patient, with the basic universally needed skills being included in all programmes. Athletes who use their vision effectively see things more quickly, more accurately and show good overall performance. Children can understand more of what they read, remember it for longer periods of time and read faster with less effort if they have good visual abilities. Great benefits can be seen in many areas of life like sports, work and learning when the processing of visual information is improved.

If a student has specific needs, new training activities can be designed to meet them.

Vision Therapy

When the visual system works more efficiently, more information can be received, processed and understood. Vision therapy, or vision training, provides a way for children to learn more efficient manners in which to use the visual system. This involves developing good body bilaterality, hand-eye coordination, form perception, directionality and visualisation skills, as well as ensuring that the muscles which focus and direct the eyes are functioning efficiently. If a child has difficulties with understanding vision input and visual perception, techniques of vision training can help them to achieve their full potential.

All of these words and phrases will make more sense as you move through the therapy programme, if vision training is necessary.

Who Can Help?

In order to establish if there may be a visual component to the learning difficulty, a full eye examination must be carried out by an optometrist. Every possible source of support will obviously have to be explored if a child has learning difficulties.

Your optometrist may choose to deal with the issue personally if a developmental visual problem is suspected (i.e. if the parts aren't coordinating properly but appear to be present and healthy). You may, however, choose to obtain a referral to a behavioural optometrist if they seem to have more experience working with learning difficulties.

What Am I Looking For?

Students who struggle to follow lines of print or keep their spot when reading may well benefit from vision training.

In many cases, mathematical ability and intelligence may be normal or higher than normal for the age, yet reading presents a problem. Often, such students will move their whole head when reading instead of just their eyes, and need a marker or finger held under the line they're reading.

Time spent reading will come to an abrupt halt and a sudden complete lack of interest. A young person with a poorly developed visual system is likely to have a very short concentration span.

Where Can I Look?

A register of all optometrists who are specifically trained in vision therapy and behavioural optometry is maintained by the British Association of Behavioural Optometrists.

What Have We Learned?

- As mysterious as vision training and the Dunlop Test may sound, they're really just ways of training eyes to respond to the correct treatment and testing the eyes fully.

- Vision training can be a tremendous help to the child if it is successful.

- These tests are usually carried out in optometrist departments in hospitals rather than at your local opticians.

- This treatment may take a few months or several years.

20

Health and Nutrition

Many scientific studies have shown that a nutritionally complete diet is necessary in the development of vision, learning ability and coordination. It's widely accepted that our children's physical and mental development rely on access to a balanced diet. One study indicated that children who had a decent breakfast before exams performed much better than those who skipped breakfast or just had a bowl of cereal.

The question is, should children be taking supplements or are they getting everything they need? And are supplements for things like zinc, iron and fatty acids capable of curing dyspraxia, ADHD and dyslexia? Loads of parents out there claim that using supplements is the only way to go, and supporting evidence is finally starting to appear.

Studies have also found that children who eat Mars bars right before exams also tend to perform slightly better. It's likely that the reason for these results is a quick surge in blood glucose levels that boost brain functioning, provided by the chocolate or the balanced breakfast.

Should We Take Supplements?

Supplements can be a safe and effective way of ensuring children are getting the nutrients needed to help them keep healthy and aid their mood and concentration generally. As a general rule, people agree that children will be well and healthy without the use of supplements if they're eating a balanced diet. Sadly, though, it's not always possible to make sure that our kids are getting all of the nutrients they need when we're constantly rushing around trying to balance every aspect of our busy lives.

Iron Supplements

An American group of scientists published a study in November 1996 which concluded that teenage girls provided with iron supplements "improved". Animal research has also hinted that iron deficiency is enough to change brain iron levels, which in turn alter the way neurotransmitters behave in the brain. Research existing prior to this also showed that the mental abilities of children was affected by anaemia.

Fatty Acids

There's further information on the link between fatty acids and ADHD in chapter X. Over the last decade, multiple studies have included that abnormal fatty acid levels in the brains of children with dyspraxia, ADHD and developmental dyslexia could be the cause of certain behavioural and practical issues.

Some parents have now seen incredible results by giving fatty acid supplements to their children with dyspraxia, ADHD and dyslexia. This does not appear to help everyone but is certainly worth trying.

Many parents have claimed that their child has very quickly become better at concentrating, calmer, and able to catch up on some writing and reading.

Michael – nine years

Dyslexic and ADHD

How Long Will I Have to Wait for the Fatty Acids to Start Working?

Two of the products containing fatty acids are:

- Soft chews: Equazen Eye Q. This product contains DHA and EPA, long chain polyunsaturated fatty acids. Long chain polyunsaturated fatty acids play an important role in the development of the eye and brain, especially vision, coordination, memory and concentration. They also include GLA from pure evening primrose oil and EPA-rich marine oil.

- Liquid or tablets: Efalex. According to the product's creators, Efamol, this is "is the only fatty acid formula that has been clinically proven to relieve symptoms of learning and behaviour disorders such as dyslexia, dyspraxia and attention deficit hyperactivity disorder". The product aims to help the development of vision and maintain eye function by providing vital long chain fatty acids, AA and DHA.

They can be purchased from chemists, health shops and most large supermarkets. In most cases, it's a good idea to start with a high dose and slowly reduce them, as it can take up to three months for fatty acids to start helping.

Fatty acid supplements can now be accessed as tablets, "chews" and liquids, so children can take them more easily.

Zinc

Research has shown that people with dyslexia can be linked with a deficiency of one of the body's most important trace minerals – zinc.

An indicator of a lack of zinc includes white marks on fingernails and dandruff. This mineral plays a vital role in the immune system of the human body. It's vital that we get enough zinc every day if we want to stay healthy, as our body won't store it even though a shortage can affect its healing process.

You can get zinc from any number of different foods, such as...

- Lean meat;
- Cheddar cheese;
- Eggs;
- Wholegrain cereals;
- Fish;
- Dried beans;
- Wholemeal breads;
- Chicken;
- Liver.

There are plenty of things that can block or break down zinc, such as food colourings, additives and tannin (found in alcohol, coffee and tea).

What Have We Learned?

- The importance of vitamin supplements is still up for debate, with experts on the subject constantly disagreeing with each other.

- Without any concrete evidence and guidance from the government, the decision has to be left to you.

- Some parents claim that children who are deficient in certain parts of their diet will make faster progress with vitamin supplements.

- Some argue that if our children receive a well-balanced diet, they do not need to take vitamin supplements.

21

The Equality Act 2010

As of October 2010, the "Equality Act" is law, aiming to support progress on equality issues by clarifying and reinforcing existing discrimination law. The Act, includes a new protection from discrimination arising from disability. It replaces and combines most of the legislation that existed prior to its introduction (e.g. the Disability Discrimination Act 1995) so that the things you need to do to comply with the law and make sure your workplace is fair are consistent.

The Equality Act states that treating a disabled person negatively as a result of their disability (e.g. if they keep making spelling mistakes because of their dyslexia) is discrimination. This type of discrimination is only justifiable if an employer can show that it is a proportionate means of achieving a legitimate aim. If the employer or their agent knows that the person has a disability, this type of discrimination is considered unlawful.

By understanding the condition you will be able to support your dyslexic employees. You need to understand the exact nature of dyslexia if you want to get the best from your staff.

Equality Act – What's New for Employers?

"Equality Act – What's new for employers", is a useful guide to help individuals and companies understand what discrimination issues mean and looks at employees' rights. This is the act you need to familiarise yourself with in order to comply with the law and provide your employees with a fair workplace environment.

The Advisory, Conciliation and Arbitration Service (ACAS) provide companies with some helpful training courses. Further information is available on the ACAS website **www.acas.org.uk**. They're here to provide you with the guidance you need to keep your business running smoothly.

What Is Dyslexia?

10% of the population have dyslexia, and 4% have severe dyslexia. Many people with dyslexia are extremely bright in lots of ways, always talking and asking questions, but they do not seem to reach their full potential in the academic field. The issues arising from this condition can impact writing, short-term memory, visual processing, coordination, number work and reading.

Things like spatial awareness, interpersonal skills and timekeeping can also be difficult. We gave a more detailed description of dyslexia in Chapter Three: Specific Learning Difficulties – Dyslexia.

What Proportion of Your Customers and Staff Have Dyslexia?

Sometimes just minor adjustments in the workplace can make it easier for your staff. Do you know what dyslexia is and how you can make "reasonable adjustments" to help those who are dyslexic? Do you know how many of your employees have dyslexia? You can support your staff more fully if you understand what dyslexia means to them. About 10% of the population are affected by dyslexia. This means it's pretty likely that it's affecting 10% of your staff, suppliers, couriers, customers and just about everyone else you know.

How Can I Make My Workplace User-Friendly?

Many dyslexics do not need a lot of adjustments to their working environment but often small changes can really help. As an employer you can help by:

- Allowing potential employees to apply for your jobs online;

- Keeping things easy-to-read by using fonts like 12pt Arial;

- Having the important information on documents highlighted;

- Using pastel coloured paper wherever possible;

- Making application forms easy. (Why not get a dyslexic employee to help design/change one or ask for help from a dyslexia charity?)

It's good practice to try and build a "user-friendly" workplace. A lot of the changes you should make are inexpensive and really easy.

There are also some handy changes you can make on computers, such as…

- Thinking about whether an employee would work better with a tablet or a laptop;

- Allowing and encouraging your employees to increase the font size if they find it helpful;

- Making sure that grammar and spelling checkers are installed on all computers;

- Using reminders on computers for important meetings, etc.;

- Using speech-to-text software;

- Making sure you can change the background colour on the screen.

Generally in the workplace:

- Try to replace memos with voice mail;

- Remind employees of important dates using large signs and boards;

- Keep the room quiet and away from distractions.

Other gadgets that can come in handy might include…

- Electronic organisers;

- Dictaphones;

- Talking calculators (really useful to people who struggle with numbers);

- Tape recorders;

- Palmtop computers.

If you can't afford some of the necessary changes, such as expensive voice-activated computers, the government's Access to Work (AtW) scheme may be able to provide funding.

Access to Work Scheme (AtW)

Access to Work can help you if your health or disability affects the way you do your job. Your local JobCentre Plus office will be operating the Access to Work Scheme. The scheme provides employers and employees with financial support and guidance.

Can I Get Support from the Access to Work Scheme?

This scheme may be able to pay for equipment, adapting premises or for a support worker. 100% of approved costs will be covered by Access to Work if the applicant is…

- Self-employed;
- Newly employed (has held the position for six weeks or less);
- Have people changing jobs in your company;
- Unemployed and starting a new job.

100% of approved costs will also be covered by AtW regardless of employment status if support is needed to cover…

- Support workers;
- Interview communicator support;
- Fares to work.

The employer in all of these cases has to order and pay for the products listed by AtW. Approved costs can then be claimed back off AtW.

Will an Assessment Be Necessary?

In order to avail of this scheme, you might need an occupational health assessment. The assessment will then identify and recommend areas to enable the dyslexic employee to benefit in the workplace. Once a need is identified, the Access to Work scheme can pay for part of the adjustments. You can have this arranged under the Access to Work scheme or through your local health authority (LHA).

You don't have to prove that you have dyslexia, but the assessment may be useful as it can help identify your precise needs.

Company bosses and employers will have to pay for part of any adjustment costs (between £300 and £1000), covering a minimum of 20% of any cost up to £10,000. Some companies may be able to offset this cost against tax. Companies with less than nine employees are classed as small companies and won't have to make a financial contribution.

The scheme will review your circumstances after a year to find out if any additional support is needed.

How Do I Find out If I'm Eligible?

Further information can be obtained from DirectGov, Access to Work Scheme, or from your local jobcentre. To find out if you're eligible for AtW support, you can download a form from the DirectGov website. A printable confirmation letter will be provided if you fit the criteria, and you can give this to your employer/prospective employer.

Supporting Employees with Dyslexic Difficulties

The "Code of Practice for Employers" is a great guide distributed by the British Dyslexia Association (BDA) which aims to help you better support your employees. This is an invaluable publication for all employers, particularly HR, Personnel and Occupational Health departments etc. The guide features advice on written tests, "reasonable adjustments", assessments, recruitment and the obligations of the employer.

You can buy this guide for £10 (plus p&p) from the BDA. It's also available as a PDF.

Where Can I Get Further Information?

You can get additional information from the following organisations.

- Your local JobCentre Plus office will be able to give you information on the Right to Work (RtW) scheme;
- Searching "protected characteristics" on **www.direct.gov.uk** will give you information on the Equality Act;
- The British Dyslexia (BDA) has an information pack available, "Code of Practice for Employers", for £10;
- For a leaflet to see if you are eligible to get support under the Access to Work scheme, go online and visit **www.direct.gov.uk**, search for "Access to Work scheme" or write to Disability on the Agenda.

You can find more useful contact details in the Help List at the back of this book.

Useful Assessments

Your local health authority or the Access to Work scheme will be able to carry out an occupational health assessment. This is available as several test types:

- Occupational health assessment;
- Educational psychologist's report;
- Dyslexia screening assessment (but you do not have to prove you are dyslexic).

These can really come in handy: the reports can identify specific work areas that can help them, even if the employee has never previously been diagnosed with dyslexia.

What Have We Learned?

- Not everyone will automatically know how to deal with discrimination issues: this is still very new legislation.

- However, the British Dyslexia Association (BDA) has very useful information on dyslexia and employers, so does ACAS.

- When most "reasonable adjustments" can be funded by the AtW scheme, employers really have no excuse for not running an accessible business.

22

Resources and Support

How Do I Set up a Support Group?

t is not difficult at all. There are lots of people out there who are unable to find a suitable support group near them and want to set up their own. When your child has special needs, it is easy to feel as if you are the only one in the world with difficulties. Everyone needs a little support and guidance at some point in their lives. Your problem will not be a new one.

It's important that parents are able to meet with others in similar situations to discuss their struggles and get advice and support from each other. If you're struggling with something, it's a safe bet that someone out there is struggling too.

How Do I Go About It?

Your first step needs to involve communicating with other parents to find out if this is something they'd be interested in.

- Check out your local Citizens Advice Bureau, charities or library to see if they have any resources that could come in handy.
- How often do you want to hold your meetings?
- Get in touch with the national charity to see if they can give you any support.
- Try to get a guest speaker for your first meeting from a national organisation.
- Where will your meetings be? (It might be best to hold the first meeting in a local hall.)
- Ask yourself, what exactly is needed in your area?

If you don't ask, you don't get – you can't do everything yourself! Talk to other parents and see if they'd be able to help out at all. This is one of those things that gets easier as it goes along, so don't panic if things are tricky to start off with.

Go for It!

It isn't as hard as you may think! So what's stopping you from setting up your own local support group? Don't wait until someone else does it – because they might not! If you think you'd benefit from the support of other parents, there must be other people in the same shoes.

Spread the News!

The local radio and newspapers need local news – let them know what you are doing. Don't forget local news is their business! You don't need to pay for advertisements to get the word out there. Most support groups have no advertising budget at all – why would they? Start spreading the news by email, telephone or snail mail.

Press Release

A press release is the quickest way to let the press know what you're doing. Don't worry, it's much easier than it sounds! All you're doing is writing a very simple letter which includes the most basic information about your group. For example…

Eddie Example,
20 Sample Street,
Big City, AB1 2CD.
012 3456 7890

Friday 13th July, 2018.

Press Release: Dyslexia Support Group

A meeting will be taking place in Big City Academy Hall on Wednesday 25th July at 19:00 to talk about the creation of a new Dyslexia Support Group.

A guest speaker from the British Association will be in attendance, and will be giving a talk entitled "Specific Educational Difficulties: What does it mean?"

Our goal is to set up a place where carers and parents can share support and information about local services. There will be a small entrance fee of £1.00. Tea and coffee will be served after the talks.

For more information, please contact Eddie Example.

Tel. 012 3456 7890

****

Don't forget: If you need support, there's always someone who can help you!

Last Words

If there's one thing to take away from this book, it is that early identification is key when dealing with dyslexia. You can start working towards a solution (without waiting for the child to fail!) once you've identified their learning difficulties and ruled out any illnesses.

The British Dyslexia Association is over 45 years old, but there is still a need for more public and professional recognition of the problem. By joining the British Dyslexia Association you will receive up-to-date newsletters and information about the latest ideas in the dyslexia world. Membership costs just a few pounds a year, and is well worth the investment.

Unfortunately, there is no magic cure or secret formula, but there is a lot of help and advice available. We hope we've managed to answer at least some of your burning questions about learning difficulties and dyslexia. Hopefully we've shown you how to use these resources to help your own child. We can all support things like awareness weeks, conferences and voluntary groups that spread an understanding of dyslexia.

Thank you for taking the time to read this book. We wish you all the best of luck with your journey.

Help List

A2Z
www.dyslexiaa2z.com

Maria Chivers is the founder of this website: Dyslexia A2Z, which has been operating for over a decade. In 2009, it merged with its sister site; Swindon Dyslexia Centre, (which opened in 1991).

ACAS
www.acas.org.uk

"Acas (Advisory, Conciliation and Arbitration Service) provides free and impartial information and advice to employers and employees on all aspects of workplace relations and employment law. We support good relationships between employers and employees which underpin business success. But when things go wrong we help by providing conciliation to resolve workplace problems."

Access to Work
www.gov.uk/access-to-work

If you're disabled or have a physical or mental health condition that makes it hard for you to do your job, you can:

talk to your employer about changes they must make in your workplace

apply for Access to Work if you need extra help.

ACE (Advisory Centre for Education Ltd)
www.ace-ed.org.uk

ACE Education Advice & Training, 72 Durnsford Road, London N11 2EJ

Tel: 0300 0115 142

ACE Education Advice & Training provides independent advice and information for parents on education issues in England. High quality training and consultancy services covering education law and guidance are provided to a wide range of education professionals.

Action on Hearing Loss
www.rnid.org.uk

1-3 Highbury Station Road, London N11SE

Tel: 0808 808 0123

"We're the UK's national charity helping people who are confronting life-changing deafness, tinnitus and hearing loss."

ADO (Adult Dyslexia Organisation)

www.adult-dyslexia.org

Ground Floor, Secker House, Minet Road, Loughborough Estate, London, SW9 7TP

Tel: 0207 924 9559

ADO is run by dyslexics for dyslexics and all those concerned with supporting Adult dyslexics. ADO not only advises and empowers dyslexic adults, supporting their particular needs, but also offers a range of services to the public and to professionals, service providers and policy makers.

Anything Left-Handed

www.anythingleft-handed.co.uk

"We are a group of left-handed people providing products and information to make life a bit easier for left-handers around the world and campaigning to promote awareness, acceptance and empathy for left-handers."

ARROW Tuition Ltd.

www.arrowtuition.co.uk

13 – 15 Flook House, Station Road, Taunton TA1 1BT.

Tel: 01823 324949

"A.R.R.O.W. is an acronym for Aural – Read – Respond – Oral – Write.

Aural …   The student listens to speech on headphones.
Read …   The student reads the text of the spoken material.
Respond … The student responds to the stimulus.
Oral …   The student repeats the spoken word(s)
Write …   The student writes down what is heard from the Self-Voice recording and marks their own work."

Arts Dyslexia Trust (ADT)

www.artsdyslexiatrust.org

artsdyst@aol.com

BABO (British Association of Behavioural Optometrists)

www.babo.co.uk

BABO, 1 Bergamot Drive, Meir Park, Stoke-on-Trent, ST3 7FD

Tel: 07443 569021

Register of members who are verified as having met the requirements for continuing education in behaviour optometry.

Back in Action

www.backinaction.co.uk

A portable seat wedge that converts to a writing slope. See website for office telephone numbers.

Bristol Dyslexia Centre

www.dyslexiacentre.co.uk

11 Upper Belgrave Road, Clifton, Bristol BS8 2XH

Tel: 0117 9739405

Specialist software 'Nessy' has been developed by the centre.

British Deaf Association

www.bda.org.uk

3rd Floor, 356 Holloway Road, London N7 6PA

Tel: 020 7697 4140

Contains the latest information about the deaf association and sign language. See the website for UK offices.

British Dyslexia Association

www.bdadyslexia.org.uk

Unit 6a Bracknell Beeches, Old Bracknell Lane, Bracknell, RG12 7BW.

Tel: 0333 405 4555

"The BDA is the voice of dyslexic people. We aim to influence government and other institutions to promote a dyslexia friendly society, that enables dyslexic people of all ages to reach their full potential."

British Mensa

www.mensa.org.uk

St John's House, St John's Square, Wolverhampton WV2 4AH, United Kingdom.

Tel: + 44 (0) 1902 772 771

Mensa was founded in England in 1946 by Roland Berrill, a barrister, and Dr Lance Ware, a scientist and lawyer. They had the idea of forming a society for bright people, the only qualification for membership of which was a high IQ. The original aims were, as they are today, to create a society that is non-political and free from all racial or religious distinctions.

Calibre

www.calibre.org.uk

Calibre Audio Library, Aylesbury, Bucks HP22 5XQ

Tel: 01296 432 339

Calibre Audio Library improves the quality of life for people with sight problems or other disabilities, who cannot read, print by bringing them the pleasure of reading through a free nationwide postal service of recorded books.

Children's Legal Centre

www.childrenslegalcentre.com

Coram Children's Legal Centre, Riverside Office Centre, Century House North, North Station Road, Colchester CO1 1RE

Tel: 01206 714 650

A unique, independent national charity concerned with law and policy affecting children and young people.

Citizens Advice Bureau (CAB)

www.nacab.org.uk

Check the website for details about their offices near you.

CReSTeD (Council for the Registration of Schools Teaching Dyslexic Pupils)

www.crested.org.uk

Old Post House, Castle Street, Whittington, Shropshire, SY11 4DF

Tel: 0845 601 5013

CReSTeD maintain a Register of Schools for dyslexic children.

Department for Education (DfE)

www.education.gov.uk

Ministerial and Public Communications Division, Department for Education, Piccadilly Gate, Store Street, Manchester M1 2WD, United Kingdom.

Tel: 0370 000 2288

The Department for Education is responsible for children's services and education, including early years, schools, higher and further education policy, apprenticeships and wider skills in England.

Directory of Social Change

www.dsc.org.uk

352 Holloway Road, London N7 6PA.

Tel: 0207 697 4200

Independent source of information and support to voluntary and community sectors.

Dyscovery Centre
dyscovery.southwales.ac.uk
Dyscovery Centre, Innovation House, University of South Wales, William Price Business Park, Treforest, Pontypridd CF37 1DL.

Tel: (+44) 01443 654799

The Dyscovery Centre was opened in Cardiff in 1997 by Professor Amanda Kirby in response to a lack of provision and coordination of services for children with Developmental Coordination Disorder (Dyspraxia) in the UK.

Dyslexia Action
www.dyslexiaaction.org.uk
Dyslexia Action Training and Guild, Centurion House, London Road, Staines-upon-Thames TW18 4AX.

Dyslexia Action Training Tel: 01784 222 304

Main functions are assessment and tuition in their 26 centres, and teacher training. They also carry out research and develop specialist teaching materials.

The Dyslexia Association
www.dyslexia.uk.net
Page Kirk Building, Sherwood House, 7 Gregory Boulevard, Nottingham NG7 6LB.

Tel: 0115 924 6888

"We provide support and services for dyslexic children and adults of all ages, their parents/ families, educators, employers and the wider community. Our head office is in Nottingham and we provide services primarily across the East Midlands (Nottinghamshire, Derbyshire, Lincolnshire, Leicestershire, Rutland, Northamptonshire) and neighbouring counties."

Dyslexia Association of Ireland
www.dyslexia.ie
DAI, 5th Floor, Block B, Joyce's Court, Talbot Street, Dublin 1.

Tel: 01 877 6001

Founded in 1972, the Dyslexia Association of Ireland (DAI) works with and for people affected by dyslexia, by providing information, offering appropriate support services, engaging in advocacy and raising awareness of dyslexia.

Dyslexia Foundation
www.dyslexia-help.org
24 Edward Pavilion, Alber Dock, Liverpool, L3 4AF.

Tel: 0800 077 8763

The organisation was set up in 1999 to support Dyslexic people, focusing on those who needed practical support and information in an accessible format.

Dyslexia International

www.dyslexia-international.org

Rue Washington 40, 1050 – Brussels, Belgium.

"Dyslexia International is a not-for-profit organization. We provide teacher-training programmes that embody latest scientific research to ensure that literacy is taught as effectively as possible in classrooms around the world."

Dyslexia Research Trust

www.dyslexic.org.uk

Dyslexia Research Trust, 179A Oxford Road, Reading RG1 7UZ.

Tel: 0118 958 5950

A wide range of information and research on dyslexia.

Dyslexia Scotland

www.dyslexiascotland.org.uk

Dyslexia Scotland, 2nd floor – East Suite, Wallace House, 17 – 21 Maxwell Place, Stirling FK8 1JU

Tel: 0344 800 8484

"Our mission is to inspire and enable everyone to reach their full potential."

The Dyslexia Shop

www.thedyslexiashop.co.uk

Email: hello@thedyslexiashop.co.uk

Tel: 01394 671 818

The Dyslexia Shop is a family run business based in Felixstowe, Suffolk which stocks thousands of carefully selected products to help people with Dyslexia and special educational needs / learning difficulties.

Dyspraxia Foundation

www.dyspraxiafoundation.org.uk

Dyspraxia Foundation, 8 West Alley, Hitchin, Herts, SG5 1EG.

Tel: 01462 454986

This registered charity offers help and advice on dyspraxia. Lots of publications available.

Education Otherwise

www.education-otherwise.net

PO Box 3761, Swindon, SN2 9GT

Tel: 01458 448286

Education Otherwise (EO) was formed by a small group of parents in 1977 and has evolved into a large self-help organisation which offers support and information to members.

Educational Psychologists (Association of)

www.aep.org.uk

4 Riverside Centre, Frankland Lane, Durham DH1 5TA.

Tel: 0191 384 9512

Efamol Ltd. (Efalex)

www.efamol.com

10 Aldersgate, London EC1A 4HJ, United Kingdom.

Direct Sales UK: Freephone 0800 472 5593

Suppliers of fatty acids.

The Equality Act

www.disability.gov.uk

Disability on the Agenda, Freepost, Bristol, BS38 7DE.

First-Tier Tribunal (HESC)

www.justice.gov.uk/guidance/courts-and-tribunals/tribunals/send/index.htm

First-tier Tribunal (Special Educational Needs and Disability), 1st Floor, Darlington Magistrates Court, Parkgate, Darlington DL1 1RU.

Tel: 01325 289 350

"We are part of the Health, Education and Social Care Chamber, one of 7 chambers of the First-tier Tribunal which settles legal disputes and is structured around particular areas of law."

Gamz

www.gamzuk.com

25 Albert Park Road, Malvern, Worcestershire WR14 1HW, United Kingdom.

Tel: 01684 562158

GAMZ was set up in 1993 by Bobbie Hill, while working with dyslexic learners. The games were developed with her pupils over a period of 10 years. She realised the need for simple, professionally produced learning aids. They had to be fast to set up, and quick and meaningful to play. They had to appeal to children and adults alike. She knows that teachers and parents need such resources and often do not have the time or the availability of economic printing facilities to produce them.

GL Assessment

www.gl-assessment.co.uk

1st Floor, Vantage London, Great West Road, Brentford, TW8 9AG.

Tel: 0330 123 5375

Provides specialist resources and testing equipment for special needs.

Helen Arkell Dyslexia Centre

www.arkellcentre.org.uk

Helen Arkell Dyslexia Centre, Arkell Lane, Frensham, Farnham, Surrey GU10 3BL.
Tel: 01252 792 400

A registered charity offering expert assessment and specialist tuition to anyone with dyslexia or other SpLDs.

Home Education UK

www.home-education.org.uk

Email: mike@home-education.org.uk

Hyperactive Children's Support Group (HACSG)

www.hacsg.org.uk

The Hyperactive Children's Support Group, 71 Whyke Lane, Chichester, West Sussex PO19 7PD.
Tel: 01243 539966

IANSYST Ltd.

www.iansyst.co.uk

Fen House, Fen Road, Chesterton, Cambridge, CB4 1UN.
Tel: 01223 420 101.

Catalogue available for thousands of specialist equipment, including computer software, etc.

Inclusive Technology

www.inclusive.co.uk

Riverside Court, Huddersfield Road, Delph, Oldham OL3 5FZ.
Tel: +44 (0) 1457 819790

Inclusive Technology is a leading supplier of software and hardware for people with special needs.

Independent Schools Council Information Services (ISCIS)

www.isis.org.uk

Independent Schools Council, St Vincent House, 30 Orange Street, London, WC2H 7HH.
Tel: 020 7766 7070

"IS Education Platform is an educational platform that is dedicated to helping people learn the best and become part of the elite in society. It is therefore very crucial to use this opportunity and learn so much more on education, from the high quality content that we avail on our site."

International Dyslexia Association

dyslexiaida.org

40 York Road, 4th Floor, Baltimore, MD 21204.

Tel: (410) 296-0232

"By joining our organization, you will be in the company of the world's foremost researchers, teachers, professionals, and parents dedicated to helping individuals with dyslexia, their families and those that support them."

IPSEA (Independent Parental Special Education Advice)

www.ipsea.org.uk

24-26 Gold Street, Saffron Walden, Essex CB10 1EJ.

Tel: 01799 582030

Gives free legally based advice to people about special educational needs.

Keith Holland Opticians

www.keithholland.co.uk

27 St George's Road, Cheltenham, GL50 3DT.

Tel: +44(0) 1242 233 500

Award-winning specialist eye-care team in the treatment of children with learning disabilities.

Keytools (BigKeys)

www.keytools.co.uk

HYPERTEC LTD, 2 Swangate, Charnham Park, Hungerford, Berks, RG17 0YX.

Tel: 0844 879 2282

Keytools is the Ergonomic and Assistive Technology arm of Hypertec Ltd, historically Keytools vision had been to provide computer access for everyone, working to help ensure all had the best possible equipment and resources to use their PC's, easily, safely and productively. Servicing all markets for over 19 years, Keytools was purchased and integrated into Hypertec Ltd in 2012.

LDA Living & Learning

www.ldalearning.com

Church Bridge House, Henry Street, Accrington, BB5 4EE.

Tel: 0345 120 4776

Wide selection of specialist software and products. Catalogue available.

Listening Books

www.listening-books.org.uk

Listening Books, 12 Lant Street, London SE1 1QH.

Tel: 020 7407 9417

"We are a UK charity providing a fantastic selection of high-quality audiobooks to some 50,000 people across the UK who find it difficult or impossible to read due to an illness, disability, learning or mental health difficulty. We help a wide range of organisations and individuals and provide our audiobooks on 3 easily accessible formats: through the post on MP3 CD, or downloaded and streamed online. Members can choose from a range of options to find the service that best suits their needs."

Local Government Ombudsman

www.lgo.org.uk

Find your local Ombudsman online.

Tel: 0300 061 0614

Government ombudsman to look into complaints from people about various matters.

Lucid Research Ltd.

www.lucid-research.com

GL Assessment, 1st Floor Vantage London, Great West Road, Brentford TW8 9AG.

Tel: +44 (0) 330 123 5375

Computerised testing equipment for dyslexia and visual stress.

Mental Health Foundation

www.mhf.org.uk

London office (headquarters): Colechurch House, 1 London Bridge Walk, London, SE1 2SX.

Tel: +44 (0)20 7803 1100

Information service, leaflets and publications available.

National Association for Special Educational Needs (NASEN)

www.nasen.org.uk

nasen House, 4/5 Amber Business Village, Amber Close, Amington, Tamworth, Staffordshire B77 4RP.

Tel: 01827 311500

National Deaf Children's Society

www.ndcs.org.uk

Ground Floor South, Castle House, 37- 45 Paul Street, London EC2A 4LS.

Tel: 020 7490 8656

Helps families, parents and carers to maximise their skills and abilities.

National Federation of the Blind of the UK

www.nfbuk.org

St. John Wilson House, 215 Kirkgate, Wakefield WF1 1JG.

Tel: 01924 291313

Organisation to make life easier for blind/partially blind people.

National Handwriting Association

www.nha-handwriting.org.uk

2 Moths Grace, Basingstoke, Hampshire, RG24 9FY, United Kingdom.

Tel: +44 (0)1256 464 598

The NHA is run by an executive committee of volunteers who work in their professional lives as teachers, therapists, academics or researchers. They are supported by a finance officer and an administrator who work part-time.

National Portage Association

www.portage.org.uk

Kings Court, 17 School Road, Hall Green, Birmingham, B28 8JG.

Tel: 0121 244 1807.

Portage is a home-visiting educational service for pre-school children with additional support needs and their families.

NIACE (now moved to Learning & Work)

www.learningandwork.org.uk

21 De Montfort Street, Leicester, LE1 7GE

Tel: (+44) 0116 204 4200

"We are an independent policy and research organisation dedicated to lifelong learning, full employment and inclusion. We bring together over 90 years of combined history and heritage from the 'National Institute of Adult Continuing Education' (NIACE) and the 'Centre for Economic & Social Inclusion'."

National Network of Assessment Centres

www.nnac.org

admin@nnac.org

"We currently represent the majority (approximately 70%) of DSA Assessment Centres in England and all centres in Wales. Our membership consists of a broad range of DSA assessment providers including those based in higher education institutions, private businesses and the Open University DSA service."

Pearson Assessment
www.psychcorp.co.uk
Halley Court, Jordan Hill, Oxford, OX2 8EJ, United Kingdom.
Tel: 0845 630 88 88
"At Pearson Clinical Assessment, we're committed to publishing standardised assessments and interventions that meet the needs of professionals working with children and adults in health, education and psychology settings."

Penfriend XP LTD
www.penfriend.biz
30 South Oswald Road, Edinburgh, EH9 2HG.
Tel: 0333 567 1467
Penfriend software benefits users who have dyslexia, visual impairment or physical disabilities and any condition which impairs the ability to write with a keyboard.

Potential Plus UK
www.potentialplusuk.org
Potential Plus UK, Challenge House, Sherwood Drive, Bletchley, Milton Keynes MK3 6DP.
Tel: 01908 646433
"Our aim is to enable children of all ages with high learning potential to grow in confidence, thrive and achieve social, emotional and academic fulfilment."

Pre-School Learning Alliance
www.pre-school.org.uk
50 Featherstone Street, London EC1Y 8RT.
Tel: 020 7697 2500
This national educational charity advises about pre-school and education.

Royal College of Speech and Language Therapists
www.rcslt.org
2 White Hart Yard, London, SE1 1NX.
Tel: 020 7378 1200

RNIB (Royal National Institute for the Blind)
www.rnib.org.uk
105 Judd Street, London, WC1H 9NE
Tel: 0303 123 9999
Leading charity working for blind and partially-sighted people.

SEN Books

www.senbooks.co.uk

618 Leeds Road, Outerwood, Wakefield, WF1 2LT.

Tel: 01924 871697

SEN Books is a specialist bookshop offering books on dyslexia, dyspraxia, ADHD, autism, Asperger and many more learning difficulties.

SEN Legal

www.senlegal.co.uk

Units 3-4, Forbes Business Centre, Kempson Way, Bury St Edmunds, IP32 7AR.

Tel: 01284 723952

Legal firm specialising in education law and special needs.

Sherston Software Ltd.

http://corp.sherston.com

185 Park Street London SE1 9DY

Tel: +44 (0)203 873 1333

Sherston facilitates personalised learning 24/7, supports teachers in delivering and tracking personal learning journeys and empowers children to take charge of their own learning.

SKILL

www.skill.org.uk

4th Floor, Chapter House, 18-20 Crucifix Lane, London, SE1 3JW.

Tel: 020 7450 0620

National Bureau for students with disabilities in post-16 education, promoting opportunities in training and employment across the UK.

Society for Italic Handwriting (SIH)

www.nickthenibs.co.uk/calligraphy.htm

11 Richmond Close, Butlers Road, Handsworth Wood, Birmingham B20 2NZ.

Tel: 0121-240 1719

Nick is Secretary of the Society for Italic Handwriting (SIH), a registered charity. It was founded in 1952 by Alfred Fairbank, a most notable British calligrapher, and Joseph Compton, a Director of Education in London. Its aim is to spread the practice of the Italic script.